Specialized Hydro-, Balneo-and Medicinal Bath Therapy

Specialized Hydro-, Balneo-and Medicinal Bath Therapy

Carola Koenig

iUniverse, Inc.
New York Lincoln Shanghai

Specialized Hydro-, Balneo-and Medicinal Bath Therapy

iUniverse books may be ordered through booksellers or by contacting:

iUniverse
2021 Pine Lake Road, Suite 100
Lincoln, NE 68512
www.iuniverse.com
1-800-Authors (1-800-288-4677)

ISBN-13: 978-0-595-36508-1 (pbk)
ISBN-13: 978-0-595-80941-7 (ebk)
ISBN-10: 0-595-36508-6 (pbk)
ISBN-10: 0-595-80941-3 (ebk)

Printed in the United States of America

CONTENTS

INTRODUCTORY LEVEL

General Introduction into Specialized Hydro-, Balneo-, and Medicinal Bath Therapy

"The human organism has no power to change inorganic matter into organic. It can not use inorganic matter to build up any part of the body."

"Disease expresses two natures; one is detoxification, the other is repair or mending."

—Kneipp Water Cure Monthly
—Principles of Hygeo Therapy-1944

INTRO/CHAPTER I

The Rational of Hydrotherapy

The action of water in disease is based upon its action in health! Since skin and water are the major elements in hydrotherapy, it is important to understand the structure and physiology of the skin as well as the physical properties of water.

- *Skin*

As part of the integumentary system, the skin is considered the largest organ of the body. Together with it appendages, hair, nails, sweat glands, and sebaceous glands, it forms approximately 16% of the body weight, 4.5 to 5 kg or 10 to 11 lb. It covers about 2 sq. m or 22 sq. ft in area with an average thickness of 1.4 to 4.0 mm or 0.06 to 0.16 in. One square inch of skin houses nearly 500 sweat glands, 100 sebaceous glands, 150 pressure sensors, 75 heat sensors, and 10 cold sensors surrounded by millions of cells. The skin is composed out of two layers: the epidermis as outer layer, tough, waterproof, protective and the dermis as thick inner layer providing strength and elasticity.

> *"The skin has the same basic structure in all vertebrates, including fish, reptiles, birds, mammals, and humans."*

The main function of the skin is to protect the body from injury, dehydration, intrusion of microorganisms and the potentially damaging ultraviolet rays of the sun. It helps to regulate body temperature and houses nerve receptors.

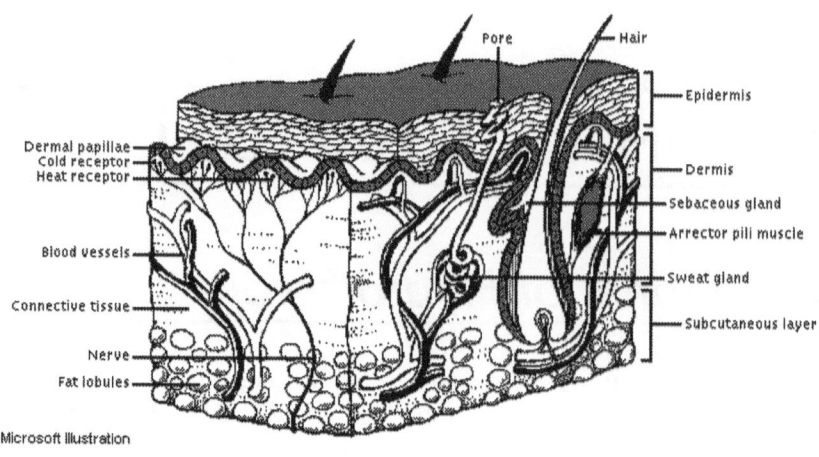

Microsoft Illustration

- *Epidermis*

Keratinocytes, which build 90% of all cells contained in the epidermis, provide the skin's protective properties. (Keratin is the main structural protein). They are arranged in layers, the stratum corneum (outer layer), here keratin replaces cytoplasma, and cells continuously move to the surface of the epidermis where they "flake off". Millions of epithelial cells are replaced daily. Cells in the inner layer of the epidermis, the stratums germinativum undergo mitosis and reproduce themselves allowing the skin to repair after injury. Melanocytes are scattered among the keratinocytes producing the pigment melanin, which is responsible for skin color and protection from the sun's ultraviolet rays. All people have roughly the same number of melanocytes. Differences in skin color result from the amount of melanin production and the arrangement of melanosomes inside keratinocytes.

Exposure to the sun causes an increase of melanin production inside the melanocytes helping to protect the skin resulting in a darkening of skin tone (suntan). The suntan fades when keratinocytes containing the extra melanin "flake off". Pheomelanin, a type of melanin dominant in "red haired" people, is responsible for their increased sensibility to sunrays.

The Langerhans cells, a type of "immune cells" produced in the bone marrow and positioned in the epidermis, help to recognize dangerous microorganism as well as chemicals. Merkel cells have contact to nerve endings in the dermis below functioning as touch receptors.

Although itself insensitive, the epidermis is capable of conveying impressions to the underlying parts.

- Dermis

In contrast to the epidermis, the dermis is supplied with an abundance of blood vessels, lymph capillaries, and a specialized network of sensory nerve endings. It is built of mainly fibrous proteins like collagen and elastin produced inside the fibroblasts, which are scattered throughout the dermis.

With age the amount of elastic fibers decreases as well as the amount of fat stored inside the subcutaneous tissue allowing wrinkles to form.

Collagen fibers account to 3/4 of the skin's weight.

The extensive network of blood vessels plays an important role in the body's temperature regulation. Nerve receptors specialized to differentiate between various stimuli, including pain, heat, cold, itch, and pressure are constantly exposed to irritation by heat and cold, which they convey to the vasomotor, respiratory, and cardiac centers as well as to muscles causing a reflectoric response.
This is the true physiologic basis of hydrotherapy, which adapts applications of cold and heat to the individual indication.
The maintenance of temperature equilibrium is one of the most important cutaneous functions.

When the body is exposed to cold temperatures the muscular structures of the skin will contract (cutis anserina-gooseflesh), blood vessels get compressed and circulation diminishes. Less heat is now lost through compression of the cutaneous vessels reducing the blood supply into the periphery and excretory glands. Cardiac action is intensified, arterial blood is driven with more force to the interior vascular area and through the muscles, enhancing their heat-producing capacity to compensate for the loss of heat at the periphery. The voluntary muscles usually respond to the demand for more heat with motion (shivering). The exposure of the body to high temperatures evokes opposite effects. The heat-regulating center in the medulla oblongata is stimulated, muscular structures of the skin relax, cutaneous vessels fill up furnishing a better blood supply to the excretory apparatus of the skin. The inner vascular area is depleted. The cutaneous glands secrete freely (perspiration) the blood is "cooled" and the body temperature is reduced.

Comparing the similarity in anatomic structure of the skin and the glomeruli of the kidneys, as well as the chemical resemblance of perspiration and urine, it is understandable that the skin is an indispensable aid to the kidneys.

Sweat glands can secrete up to 10 liters or 2.6 gallons of fluid per day. Sebaceous glands are found all over the body except on the palms, the soles, and the top of the feet. They produce sebum, which protects the skin and hair from drying out and inhibits bacteria growth. Wax or ceruminous glands inside the ear canal protect the ear from foreign particles.

Keratin filled epidermal cells form fingernails and toenails, which protect the digits from injury.
The nail body appears pink because of blood circulating in the tissue underneath its base, the semi-circular lunula is pale, due to the thick layer of epidermal cells without blood vessels.
Fingernails grow 1 mm or 0.04 inches per week, hair on the scalp grows approximately 1 mm or 0.04 inches every three days.
The hair color is determined by melanin incorporated into the keratinocytes, which form the hair. Dark hair contains pure melanin. White, blond, and red hair result from types of melanin containing sulfur and iron.

Generally substances enter systemic circulation directly through the skin's surface in a dissolved solution, which diffuses into extra cellular fluids and than through the extremely thin walls of lymph vessels and capillaries.

- *Lymphatic System*

The Lymphatic System builds the major part of the body's immune defenses; it fights against infectious pathogens, like bacteria and viruses, it collects interstitial fluids and filters out impurities. Lymph is formed when high arterial pressure forces fluid out of the capillaries into the tissue spaces. From there it is taken up into the lymphatic vessels.

- *Anatomy/Physiology*

Like the Venous System, the Lymphatic System builds a Superficial System and a deeper system consisting of larger vessels. The Superficial System builds a network of valveless lymph capillaries covering the entire body (60,000 miles of capillaries) the deeper lymph vessels are formed by little segments called Lymphangions, which are separated by one-way valves allowing the lymph to flow in one direction towards the nearest filter station made of lymph nodes. Valves prevent backflow of lymph.

As a number of lymph vessels decreases towards the center of the body, their size in diameter increases (thoracic duct). On its way through the body, the lymph fluid is cleansed and concentrated by passing through regional lymph nodes arranged in groups or chains. There are approximately 600 lymph nodes throughout the body. Form and size of lymph nodes vary between 2mm and 25mm. Lymphocytes are able to migrate throughout the lymphoid tissues and circulate between different organs via lymphatic channels.

The Lymphatic System interacts with the Circulatory System acting as a filter and drainage network. Arteries transport oxygenated blood, plasma, and nutrients towards every single cell. The Venous System reabsorbs 90% of the deoxygenated/carbon dioxide rich fluid and metabolic waste, 10% remain as lymph obligatory load. The heart pumps blood under pressure though the arterial and venous system. Lymph is only circulated by muscle contraction. The human body consists of approximately 70% water.
We distinguish between:

- ❑ Intra cellular fluid (inside the cell)
- ❑ Extra cellular fluid (surrounding the cells)
- ❑ Interstitium or interstitial spaces
- ❑ Interstitial fluid

The interstitial fluid serves as food supplier and garbage dump at the same time. Minerals and vitamins are supplied and cell residue and metabolic waste is reabsorbed.

Lymphostasis

The correct function of lymphangions can be hindered or stopped due to fatigue, stress, emotional shock, severe colds, infections, lack of mobility, chemicals, and food additives causing lymphostasis. Which means lymph circulation stagnates, fluids, proteins, hormones, fatty acids, immune cells as well as toxins accumulate and cellular functioning is comprised. Long-term lymphostasis can also affect the liver, lungs, and intestines. Which will lead to dysfunction or even damage of the specific organs.

Lymph Edema

Ignored lymphostasis will lead to lymph edema. Untreated lymph edema is progressing. Protein rich interstitial fluid will be replaced by fibrotic tissue causing low oxygen tension and severe secondary infections (erysipelas/cellulite). Lymph edema is a malfunction or insufficiency of the lymphatic transport capacity for several reasons:

> cancerous and non-cancerous tumors, surgical or non-surgical scar formation due to normal wound healing, radiation, or chemotherapy. Even minor disturbances in the micro circulation of the connective tissue can result in congestion and edema. It is essential to differentiate the cause of swelling, location, leading lymph vessels, and lymph nodes (troubleshooting).

- Lymph nodes may swell to block access for bacteria/virus towards vital organs.

- Lymphatics may swell to protect trunk from invasions of allergens (sinus, tonsils, neck)

- Lymphostasis of the face, e.g. may be the result of adhesion formed by scarring after accidents, injuries, surgeries, and radiation of sublingual lymph nodes. Relieving congestion and lymph edema through manual lymph drainage has been scientifically proven to prevent pathology.

- *Neuro-Lymphatic Reflexes/Chapman's Reflexes*

  The Neuro-lymphatic Reflex correlates to the Sympathetic Nervous System. Whenever the neuro-lymphatic reflexes are blocked, the Sympathetic Nervous System is overloaded.

  Extreme or continuous stress causes "sympathetic dominance", or adrenal exhaustion, which weakens the body's immune defenses. The lymphatic system becomes impaired, lymphatic drainage blocks and metabolic waste accumulates.

  Neuro-lymphatic reflexes are known as switches, which can promote lymph-flow changes via the sympathetic and spinal nerves.

  Neuro-lymphatic reflex-points of the liver are mostly found anterior and posterior to the intercostal spaces. The stimulation of the Neurolymphatic reflexes can help the body to "turn on" the mechanism to aid the lymph flow. Even though it is not the lymph flow, which brings about the change, it is the stimulation of a specific communication system that activates a whole series of impulses, which "unblock" (remove static) and allow the body to communicate more effectively.

During detoxification therapy, it is most important to assure that the excretion of toxins from the superficial, the deep, and the intermediate tissue layers is balanced. The removal of toxins from the tissues should never be faster than the possible elimination, to avoid unpleasant reactions.

Nervous System

Through conduction paths, emotions are able to affect, even change, autonomic functions. Stress, anger, and fear lead to increased sympathetic activity. Internal organs are mostly influenced by the autonomic nervous system; they receive parasympathetic and sympathetic impulses.

- For instance the heart beats faster through sympathetic impulse whereas parasympathetic impulses slow it down but increase peristalsis of the colon and the production of insulin or digestive enzymes.

- The body does not metabolize protein very well under heavy stress, protein will excrete as amino acid in urine.

- Skin temperature correlates with blood flow in organs via dermatomes. (If skin over the heart region feels colder, then blood circulation in heart impaired same for liver and kidney)
The Autonomic Nervous System was discovered in 1890. The principle of the "lie detector" is based upon autonomic nervous responses.
   The detector measures the resistance of the skin to an electric current. Moisture in the skin is regulated by the sympathetic nervous system. Moist skin is more conductive to electric currents.

A nerve impulse is a specialized electrical stimulation associated with and triggered by chemical changes. Simply a nerve impulse at the axon causes the discharge of neurotransmitters into the synapse. Neurotransmitter molecules than interact with specific receptors on the membranes of dendrites. This interaction changes the electrical activity of the neuron, causing it to become excited. Consequently, either a muscle cell contracts or a glandular cell manufactures and secretes a hormone. The response time varies from one second to several hours. The behavioral effects of many drugs and neurotoxins have been linked with their ability to disrupt or modify neurotransmitters. Human nerve impulses travel at a speed of 3 to 300 feet per second. Speed and intensity remain constant all along the nerve fibers and are not influenced by the intensity of the stimulus that started the impulse. However, stronger or repeated stimuli affect more fibers, which increases the frequency of the impulses resulting in a stronger response.

The nervous system can be divided in two main parts. The central nervous system consisting of brain and spinal cord which stores and processes information and sends messages to muscles and glands. The peripheral nervous system consisting of twelve pairs of cranial nerves located in and near the medulla oblongata and thirty-one pairs of spinal nerves. (8 cervical, 12 thoracic, 5 lumbar, 5 sacral nerves, and 1 coccyx nerve)

The cranial Nerves:

1.) Olfactory Nerve	conducts from *nose to brain*	⇨sense of smell
2.) Optic Nerve	conducts from *eye to brain*	⇨vision
3.) Oculomotor N.	conducts from *brain to eye muscles*	⇨eye movements
4.) Trochlear N.	conducts from *brain to external eye muscle*	⇨eye movements
5.) Trigeminal N.	conducts from *skin, mucos-membrane, teeth*	⇨face, teeth, chewing
6.) Abuducens N.	conducts from *brain to external eye muscle*	⇨eye movement
7.) Facial N.	facial muscles, salivary glands	⇨taste, facial expression
8.) Vestibulocochlear	from *ear to brain*	⇨hearing, balance
9.) Glossopharyngeal	from *tongue* to *brain, brain to head*	⇨taste, swallowing
10.) Vagus	main nerve of the parasympathetic nervous system	
11.) Accessory	*brain* to *neck, shoulder muscle*	⇨swallowing, moving head/shoulder
12.) Hypoglossal	from brain to tongue	⇨tongue muscles

Types of Receptors and Their Functions

Chemoreceptors	taste buds, cilia in nasal cavity	Detect chemicals in food and air
Mechanoreceptors	Cilia in ear	Detect movement of ear drum and ossicles (ear bones)
Osmoreceptors	Hypothalamus	Detects concentration of solutes in the bloodstream
Photoreceptors	Retina of eye	Detect light
Proprioceptors	Muscles	Detect positioning and movement of limbs
Stretch Receptors	Lungs, tendons, Ligaments	Detect expansion or elongation of muscle tissue

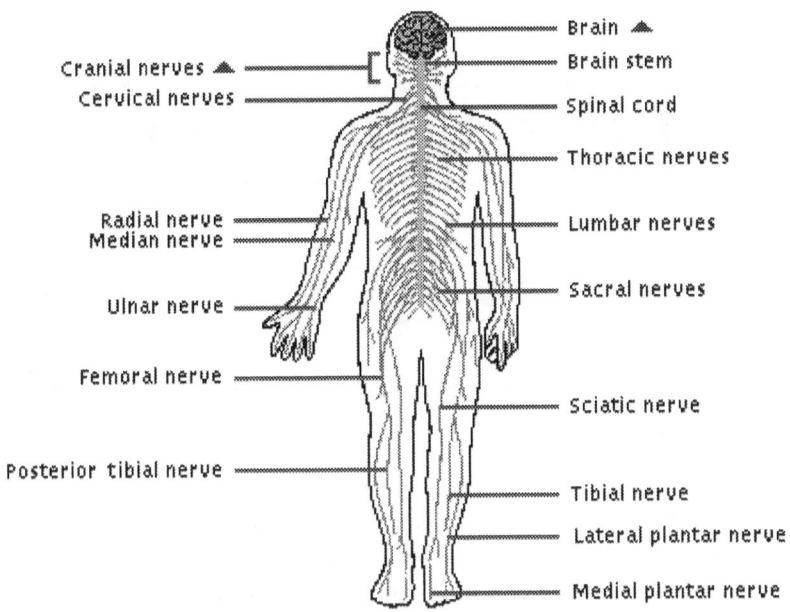

Brain ▲

Cranial nerves ▲

Brain stem

Cervical nerves

Spinal cord

Thoracic nerves

Radial nerve
Median nerve

Lumbar nerves

Ulnar nerve

Sacral nerves

Femoral nerve

Sciatic nerve

Posterior tibial nerve

Tibial nerve

Lateral plantar nerve

Medial plantar nerve

Intro/Chapter II

Physics of Water

> "Water is one part oxygen, two parts hydrogen and the rest is magic"
> C.S. Lewis

Water is considered the "universal solvent" because it dissolves more substances than any other liquid. Wherever water goes, either through the ground or through our bodies, it takes along valuable chemicals, minerals, and nutrients. Pure water has a neutral pH level 7, neither acidic nor basic.

Water is also unique for being the only natural substance found in three stages.

1.) Liquid ⇨ water
2.) Solid ⇨ ice
3.) Gas ⇨ steam

The form of the water depends on the temperature and pressure. Melting ice requires heat. This heat is chemically used to break the hydrogen bonds, which tend to hold the ice in a solid form. Boiling water requires even more heat to overcome hydrogen bonds in the liquid state. This additional heat is referred to as latent heat of evaporation.

Water freezes at 32 F or 0 Celsius and boils at 212 F or 100 Celsius at sea level, at 14,000 feet elevation it boils at 186.4 F. Salt water freezes at 1.9 C and boils at 100.5 C. The density of ice is lower than the liquid stage of water, which explains why ice floats on water. If ice would sink to the bottom soon after its formation, a lake would freeze from the bottom up, which would eradicate marine life.

As a matter of fact, the floating ice cover on a lake is insulating the water underneath from the cold. The insulating capacity of ice limits the thickness of the "ice blanket" at the surface.

The density of seawater is controlled by temperature and salinity.

1.) increased salinity causes increased density.

2.) decreasing temperature causes increased density.

Due to its high specific heat index water is able to absorb a lot of heat before it gets hot.

> The high specific heat index of water also helps to regulate temperature changes in the air especially near the oceans. Biogeochemical cycles in the ocean like the onshore/offshore wind patterns near the coast are direct results of the waters higher heat capacity in relation to the land.

Water is an excellent conductor with the unique ability to absorb and transfer large amounts of heat easily. This heat is defined as kinetic energy; it can be transferred to a body surface by conduction, convection, or conversion.

Heat is transferred via *conduction* during applications like: fomentation, hot bath, hot pack, hot shower, etc.
A heat-transfer via *convection* occurs as steam moves in currents around the body (Sauna, Russian Steam Bath).
Therapies like ultrasound, diathermy, or infrared transfer heat as energy into the body via *conversion*.
The capacity for conducting heat is 27 times higher in water than in air.

Water is inexpensive in essence and easily available as a therapy tool. Generally the impact of application is determined by temperature, duration (length), and the body area immersed in or exposed to water. Chemical factors such as botanical extracts, salts, or seaweed are also important variables.

Exploring the dimensions of water application is the first step towards "Natural Health".

Hydrotherapy:
is the use of water with dietetic, prophylactic, or therapeutic purpose in all thermal stages from steam to ice application.

Balneotherapy:
is the therapeutic application of bath (partial-, half-, full-) with or without herbal or mineral extracts, gas, peloids, mud & clay.

Including drinking of mineral water or inhalation. Balneology is the science of water application and knowledge about the physiological impact, as well as medicinal uses of mineral and thermal waters. Crenology strictly refers to healing springs and mineral water. Climatology deals with weather related factors affecting the function of the human body.

Medicinal Bath Therapy distinguishes three categories
   1.) synthetic medicinal bath
   2.) bath with phytoextracts
   3.) specialized medicinal baths
       Four-cell bath (Hydroelectric bath), colon hydrotherapy

Important factors in Hydrotherapy

- *Temperatures*
  impact all physiological and chemical reactions in the human body especially the heat regulating centers and the vasculatory system
- *Hydrostatic Pressure*
  surrounds the submerged body equally and affect respiration and blood circulation
- *Buoyancy (buoyant effect)*
  appears to reduce the weight of the submerged body equal to the weight of the water displaced. It decreases muscle tension and allows a better mobility.

> The "Archimedes Principle" states: that the force acting to buoy up a body partially or totally immersed in water is equal to the weight of the water displaced.
>
> Archimedes (287-212 B.C.)
> Greek mathematician, also founded
> the science of hydrostatics.

The buoyant force opposes the force of gravity that pulls the body downward. By diminishing the effects of gravity stress on joints is reduced and allows easier movement.
- *Force of Resistance*
  is mostly taken advantage of by muscle strengthening exercises. With increased motion resistance will equally increase.

- *Mechanic Factors*
  are considered additional stimuli intentionally provoked by brushing or underwater jets.
- *Chemical Factors*
  offer additional benefits through minerals naturally present in spring or seawater or added by specific bath extracts.

All these factors act in conjunction with each other increasing the effectivity of the determined treatment protocol accomplishing pronounced effects on the vasculatory system, the nervous system, muscles, metabolism, leukocytes, immune system, endocrine, basically all tissues and organs.

To give an example for the interaction of different factors lets look at a seawater bath, which offers a <u>chemical</u> component based upon the salt contents, the <u>mechanical component</u> comes from the hydrostatic pressure and waves, whereas the <u>thermic</u> component is based upon the temperature of water and air. If the seawater bath is now taken outside in the ocean the already comprehensive impact maybe increased by exercise against a high level of resistance (wind + waves + hydrostatic pressure) and if the sun is shining we experience an additional factor of ultraviolet light.

Sunlight is known to

- have a regulative effect on the vegetativum
- improve the recovery from strenuous work or illness
- have antibacterial effects
- have an antirachitic effect through the development of vitamin D
- raise or regulate calcium levels

In order to explain the impact of the hydrostatic pressure on coronary functions, breathing, and circulation, I will give a few examples.

1.) If a person is standing in water up to the inguinal area the venous backflow from the legs is supported; are additional muscle contracting exercises applied the benefits will increase because of the internal pressure.

2.) If the person is now standing in chest high water, the venous backflow is now increased back to the heart. Diaphragm is pushed upward after exhalation. Inhalation requires slightly more effort.

3.) Standing in water up to the neck will impact the heart and all blood vessels as well as lymph vessels. The pressure upon the chest supports exhalation and forms a resistance training for all tissues involved in inhalation.

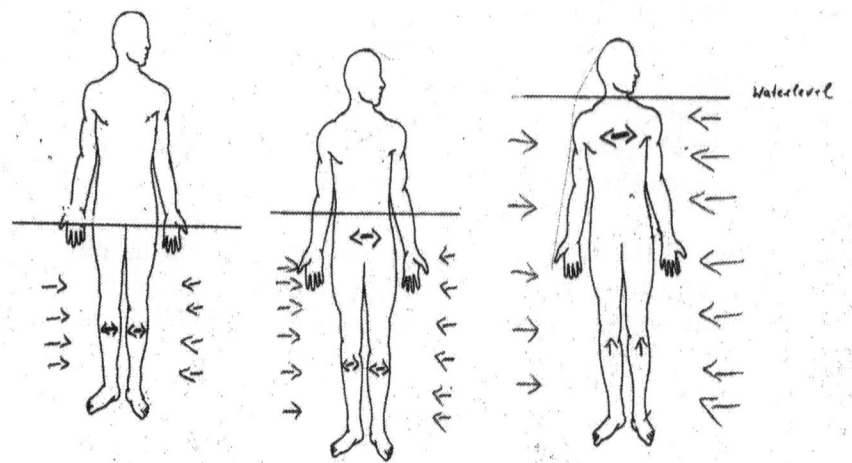

Different Water Levels

Even though the pressure is experienced as minimal it can create problems for vasolabile people. With increased water temperature, chances for fainting increase as well, especially by exiting the pool or even bathtub. By leaving the water the external pressure disappears very sudden whereas the blood vessels remain dilated and an immediate loss in blood pressure occurs. (blackout) This is a perfect example for counteracting effects due to temperature.

Hydrostatic ⇨ pressure + cold water = compression + vasoconstriction muscle is forced to work harder to maintain circulation.

Hydrostatic pressure + warm water = compression + Vasodilation* = eases blood circulation due to enlarged vessel volume.

Neither one is recommended for patients with coronary problems!

Treatment of disease using water (hydrotherapy) is a very important part of physiotherapy. Water can be used internally (drinking of mineral water) and externally in many ways to suit a specific condition. The application of water can produce various physiologic reactions in the circulatory as well as the nervous system.

Intro/Chapter III

Physiology of Hot and Cold Triggers

The temperature variation is one of the most important tools in hydrotherapeutic application. The temperature of the water determines the extent on stimulation via the skin receptors to the nervous system. Sensory receptors are more aware of temperature changes than of absolute temperature. As an example take a look at the contrast hot and cold footbath.

For our little demonstration: place one foot into a bucket with 90 F water and the other one into a bucket with 40 F water. After 2 minutes put both feet into a bucket with 70 F water. The foot that dipped in 90 F water will experience the 70 F cold whereas the other from the 40 F water will sense the 70 F as hot. So each foot has a different thermic impression even though they are in the same temperature. It is very important to keep in mind that profound physiological changes can occur inside the body just by shifting the temperature of the water used for a specific treatment a few degrees up or down. There are several reflexive connections between the skin receptors of specific areas of the body and the vascular system of certain remote organs. By altering the temperature of hands and feet the circulation in pelvis, chest, and head is influenced. For example, if a cold compress is applied to abdomen or back, the blood vessels of the pia mater dilate widely after a brief contraction.

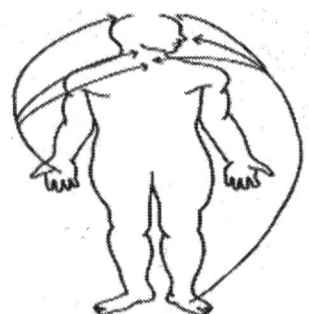 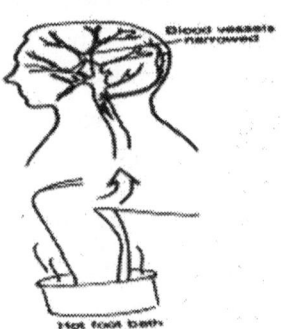

Vasoconstriction response to a hot and cold bath

The application of a hot footbath will cause a narrowing of cranial blood vessels relieving pressure or congestion intracranially. This reaction of contracting vessels at a distance and dilating vessels locally is referred to as derivation. By contracting cranial blood vessels, blood is transferred from the head to another part of the body.

The most intense form of derivation is obtained by a combination of hot and cold. By applying a hot blanket pack to legs and hips plus an cold compress to the pelvis we force the spinal nerves to mediate the reflex which contracts the blood vessels in the uterus and dilates the blood vessels in the skin.

Metabolic action is also influenced by hydrotherapy. Cold applications briefly increase the elimination of carbon dioxide (CO_2) and shifts then to a reduction of CO_2 elimination. Alkalinity of the blood favors the actions of leukocytes whereas acidosis inhibits those. Carbonic acid occurs by transferring CO_2 from the tissues to the lungs. Hyperventilation triggered by hydrotherapy reduces carbonic acid consequently alkalizing the blood favoring phagocytosis.

Brief Cold Application in Contrast to Prolonged Cold

- very brief cold application to face, hands, and head increases mental alertness (spray or gush)
- to the chest (above the heart) increases heart pulse rate
- brief cold shower (gush) for 30 seconds after hot shower will cause a general peripheral vasoconstriction

▸ prolonged cold application to the skin in abdominal region causes increased intestinal blood flow with increased intestinal activity and increased gastric acid production.

▸ prolonged cold to hands and skin of the scalp causes contraction of intracranial blood vessels.

▸ prolonged cold in acute trauma like contusions and sprains causes a vasoconstriction and lessens pain, swelling, and hemorrhage into tissue

Two specific rules apply for cold applications.

    1.) the person must be "warm" (not shivering)

    2.) the room temperature must be at least 70 F (normal body temperature 98.6 F.)

General Physiological reaction:
Cold at fist causes an active vasoconstriction producing paleness, goose bumps, and a shiver with a dilation of internal blood vessels after a brief contraction. Derivation causes the maximum possible dilation of cutaneous blood vessels after 5-8 minutes. (capillary constriction induced by cold lasts five to eight minutes after termination of the cold treatment)
A sensation of warmth occurs with reduced pulse rate and increased blood pressure.

The application of "cold" creates two responses:

1.) the primary "action" locally (capillary vasoconstriction) and

2.) a secondary "reaction" due to the reflectoric responses in internal organs as result to the cold application to the surface.

The consequences of a thermic application can be the vasoconstriction at a distance and a dilation of vessels locally based on intensity and duration.
A hot footbath for instance will constrict blood vessels inside the head, relieving intracranial pressure and congestion. (without primary dilation) In contrast a warm or hot compress applied to the feet triggers the narrowing of cranial blood vessels secondarily after the primary brief dilation!

If we combine the primary and reflexive responses we receive a very important tool. For example, to relief a congestive headache: apply a hot footbath together with a cold compress to the head the neck. (derivation +brief retrostasis shifting to derivation)

The primary action of cold is to drive blood to the interior ⇨ retrostasis.

The primary action of heat draws blood to the surface ⇨ derivation.

Remember cold has a secondary reflexive reaction to the primary retrostasis!
⇨ Derivation (just like it occurs after heat)

Now lets investigate the hot blanket pack to hips and legs combined with a cold pack to the pelvis. Through skin receptors, the spinal nerves try to mediate the responsive vasoconstriction taking place in the uterus and dilate the subcutaneous blood vessels.

Retrostasis eventually turns to derivation (cold to pelvis) + dilated subcutaneous blood vessels as result to the hot blanket pack (derivation as heat response) throughout the legs, = optimal circulation to the uterus relieving congestion, inflammation.

- *Effects of Heat applications:*

The vascular dilation due to heat is passive. The application of heat is initially an excitant, which turns to be a depressant later on. All heat applications lower the alkalinity of the blood within the area treated. The increased respiration causes the excretion of alkaline substances via the kidneys, creating an elevation of urinary pH. The diuresis is primary associated with the bath, the temperature appears to have the lesser impact.

The blood pressure shows a variety of different responses to different degrees of heat. The diastolic pressure decreases with a mild warm bath due to the dilation of subcutaneous capillaries. The systolic pressure starts to increase quite drastic with a hot (98-105 F) bath but moderate elevation of diastolic pressure as well. Consequently, hot baths should be avoided in patients with heart disease and circulatory problems.
A moist heat application causes profuse perspiration, eliminating toxins, lactic acid, uric acid, creatinine phosphates and sulfates and certainly a loss of water. It causes the elevation of body temperature but a decrease in blood pressure. The metabolism accelerates and the amount of white blood cells increases.

Whenever profuse sweating occurs during heat application or during the resting time after the treatment, a quick shower is indicated to remove toxic materials from the surface of the skin to avoid autointoxication.

As mentioned in chapter one, substances, directly enter systemic circulation through the skin. Substances readily absorbed include oxygen, carbon dioxide, fat solubles, vitamins, steroids, plant resins like poison oak or poison ivy, paint thinners, and heavy metal salts.

The temperature in heat treatments should be raised slowly; a quick application will cause an immediate vasoconstriction.

A controlled response can occur to adjust temperature-regulating mechanisms in as little as one second. (A sympathetic nervous response from one hand to another, feet to hands, or one foot to the other foot).

Temperature

Since water is an excellent conductor it transfers heat quickly and effectively. It can also absorb and distribute large quantities of heat. The capacity to conduct heat is 27 times higher in water than in air. It is able to give up its heat rapidly, without cooling quickly. Because of the fact that water temperature determines the extent of skin stimulation it is an important factor in water therapy. Since one primary function of the skin is to maintain the body's temperature in order to assure homeostasis any thermal change creates a stimulus to nerve receptors transferring impulses via nerves, lymph, and blood vessels to larger organs. The body will respond by increasing or decreasing circulation therefore a natural detoxification or elimination process takes place.

Hyperthermic bath or artificial fever-baths have been used in certain cancer treatments. It is extremely important to keep the maximum tolerance temperature in mind, the highest possible temperature the body can tolerate without sustaining damage. It is 45-46 C/116-120 F in water and 100 C in the air depending on duration of exposure and percentage of exposed aerial. The tolerance temperature of a heat conductor changes proportionally: it decreases with increasing amounts of water.

Definitions of Water Temperature

Possibly injurious	50 C	Above 125 F
Painfully hot	42.8-46 C	110-120 F
Very hot	40-42.8 C	104-110 F
Hot	38-40 C	100-104 F
Neutral	34.4-37 C	94-97 F
Warm	34-38 C	92-100 F
Tepid	27-34 C	80-92 F
Cool	21-27 C	70-80 F
Cold	13-21 C	55-70 F
Very Cold	0-13 C	32-55 F

Normal Body Temperatures: Surface and Internal

Tip of Ear: 83.64	Cheek: 93.92
Breast: 88	Pectoral Region: 94.5
Back of hand: 90.5-91.76	Hollow of closed hand: 94.94
Calf: 92.5	Rectum: 100
Forehead: 93.38 to 93.92	Blood: 102

Sternum: 93.9   Brain: 104
Right iliac fossa: 93.9   Right ventricle: 106
Hollow of open hand: 93.9-94.6   Liver: 106.5
Left ventricle: 107

Burns at Specific Temperatures

Temperature	Length of Exposure	Degree of Burn
158 (70 C)	1 second	full thickness of skin
149 (65 C)	2 seconds	full thickness of skin
140 (60 C)	3.5 seconds	full thickness of skin
135 (57 C)	10 seconds	full thickness of skin
133 (56 C)	15 seconds	full thickness of skin
127 (53 C)	60 seconds	full thickness of skin
124 (51 C)	3 minutes	full thickness of skin

Special Responses to Cold and Hot

Cold

Heart: first fast, then slow
Vessels: the action, contraction, the reaction, dilation
Nerves: numbing
Muscles: reduces volume
Respiration: slows and deepens
Stomach: increases hydrochloric acid and motion
Blood: increases blood count, both RBC's (30-50%) and WBC's (15-50%); increases phagocytosis unless prolonged to chilling.
Kidneys: congests and stimulates
Metabolism: increases CO_2 in blood by increasing production of CO_2; decreases urea; improves oxidation

Hot

Heart: first slow, then fast
Vessels: the action, dilation; the reaction; contraction when intense
Nerves: excites
Muscles: increases volume
Respiration: quickens
Stomach: decreases hydrochloric acid and motion

<u>Blood:</u> increases blood count, both RBC's and WBC's increases phagocytosis

<u>Kidneys:</u> reduces activity

<u>Metabolism:</u> decreases CO_2 in the blood by over breathing; increases urea and general protein wastes.

INTRO/CHAPTER IV

Climatology

Air is a composition of one part oxygen and four parts nitrogen plus traces of argon, neon, krypton, and xenon. The air we breathe contains approximately 21 percent oxygen. The amount of nitrogen ranges around 78 percent. Of course additional impurities from dust to perfumes are unfortunately also present.

In a resting stage, a person uses 580 to 1000 litres of air. A 250-300 lbs. person performing physical work will need more than 1000 litres of air in 24 hours compared to an office worker who uses only 400 litres of air. Respiration varies from 3 breaths per minute up to 30 breaths during physical activity.

While researching hydrotherapy and Balneology the strong connection to climatology becomes obvious. (Institute of Medical Balneology and Climatology, University Munich/Germany, International Society of Medical Hydrology and Climatology) Climatology focuses mostly on air chemistry; like air pressure, winds, humidity, light, ultraviolet effects in different altitudes, and temperature in regards of impact to organs and structures of the human body. Science has proven that climatic phenomena do influence our health.

Friction of clouds, hail, snow, humidity, atmospheric pressure changes have effects on brain and circulation via the nervous system and certain people are more sensitive than others. Response may be sleeplessness and slower recuperation.

Any storm creates electrical variation and since the nervous system basically runs on electrical impulses, changes in atmospheric pressure are noticeable. Ozone is also formed during (electrical) thunderstorms. The ozone molecule (O_3) consists of 3 oxygen atoms, ordinary oxygen (O_2) consists of two oxygen atoms. Some people may experience respiratory difficulties. Eye irritation, and fatigue after an hour of exposure to ozone concentrations as low as 0.12 parts per million (ppm). People with respiratory or heart problems are extra susceptible. Ozone is formed in the upper atmosphere by ultraviolet radiation from the sun. The UV-radiation breaks the ordinary oxygen molecules apart to form ozone.

Electrical discharges like lightning or welding arcs form ozone in a similar manner.

Ozone in smog is formed as a result from chemical reactions between certain air pollutants. (Hydrocarbon compounds + nitrogen oxides +sunlight) Surprisingly electricity has also a positive effect on the soil. Lightning helps fertilize the soil by producing up to ten million tons of nitrogen annually. When lightning strikes the air, it creates nitrogen compounds, which are washed to the ground by raindrops supplying natural fertilizer. (Dr. Martin A. Uman: "Understanding Lightning") However dust, dirt, and microorganisms are also washed down with rain.

Storms are only "air in motion", warm air expands and ascends, as cold air takes it place producing air circulation (wind).

Wind at:

8 miles per hour	is hardly noticeable
13 mph	is a pleasant breeze
19 mph	gentle breeze
24 mph	moderate breeze
29 mph	fresh breeze
34 mph	medium wind
49 mph	fresh wind
56 mph	strong wind
68 mph	storm
75 mph	strong storm
88 to 150 mph	hurricane

The weight of air is considerable when we realize that 11 to 15 tons of air pressure is beating down on us constantly. The most incredible measurable effects on red blood cells are created by altitude. At sea level human blood contains about 5 million red blood cells per cubic millimeter. People at altitudes of 5000 to 6000 feet have seven to eight million red blood cells.

In the South American Andes at 10,000 to 12,000 feet people have red blood cells of 7,500,00.

Atmospheric pressure diminishes at higher altitudes and with higher pressure at lower altitudes the red blood cells are proportionally reduced.

Respiration is also affected at higher altitude. The increased expansion of chest volume increases oxygenation, metabolism is quickened and the thyroid works at a more rapid pace.

If we go too high, however, new symptoms and problems will occur.

Although people have adapted well to different climates there is a relatively narrow range of temperatures in which human life can exist comfortably and healthy because the core body temperature should be maintained at about 98.6 F (37 C).

Seasonal temperature variations are known to reflect upon health. Mortality rates are the highest in winter, with increase in circulatory, respiratory, and infectious diseases. Cold temperatures increase blood pressure and place more stress on the heart. Chilling of the body reduces the resistance to infections.

Warm temperatures on the other hand increase bacteria growth though diseases spread via food and poor sanitation.

Respiratory infections and muscular pain seem to appear with sudden changes in temperature and humidity.

Heart attacks, bleeding ulcers, and migraines have also been linked to abrupt weather changes. In hot weather, the level of heat and humidity determines the level of comfort to humans.

Humidity is invisible water vapor in the air, not snow, fog, rain, or dew. Cold air holds less humidity than hot air. The humidity decreases with increasing altitude. Moisture intensifies both heat and cold, while dry air decreases heat. During high humidity, the skin function is more active.

High temperature combined with muggy air lowers respiration and other functional activities, which consequently increases the carbon dioxide levels in blood and tissue. In colder air more carbon dioxide is exhaled due to deeper breathing. Even the effects of caffeine, alcohol, and nicotine create different responses under different climatic conditions.

The occurrence of arteriosclerosis, tuberculosis, sinusitis, and many other health problems can be linked to man-made weather. (air conditioning)

Now what does all this have to do with hydrotherapy? Just show us how to apply water!

Well, the reason for all these extensive excursions, not "directly" related to hydrotherapy, is to explain the connection of the human body to its environment. And for the therapist it could be critical to choose the right application under different circumstances.

I hate to disappoint my students if they expect me to just tell them what to do. Unfortunately, there is no "one fits all", even dealing with plain water without extracts. Just Water, we still have to decide, how long (duration), how much (half-bath, full bath, spray, mist, etc.), how warm (cold, indifferent, warm, tepid, hot).

And let me assure you once you stop falling asleep over this subject, finally you realize it is quite interesting and you will be able to transfer valuable information into different everyday situations like exercise and cold drinks for instance. Generally after a vigorous workout I see people sit down and have a cold drink. The exercise creates a state of maximum circulation throughout the body. Sitting down immediately after exercise drastically reduces the circulation to the limbs increasing therefore the blood volume to lungs, head, heart, and liver. The additional ice cold drink now causes sudden reflectoric vasoconstriction of all major internal blood vessels placing an increased burden to the vital organs. Some of the consequences can be stroke, heart attack, embolism due to sudden vasoconstriction and massive pressure.

- An ice-cold drink in a hot climate at a resting stage will cause the intestinal walls to contract and consequently impair digestion.

- Eating ice cream contracts the stomach wall, shutting down the hydrochloric acid secretion, which is needed to digest the nutritious ingredients (milk, sugar, fat).

LEVEL I/CHAPTER I

Evolution & Renaissance of Hydrotherapy

Historical Traces

People have used geothermal and mineral waters for bathing and health for thousands of years. Balneology as practice of using natural mineral spring water for the prevention and cure of disease, can be traced back about 5000 years to the Bronze Age, although there is evidence that humans have been using hot springs for more than 600,000 years.

From the dawn of recorded history, various baths have been used for pleasure and the treatment of disease. The Babylonians, the Egyptians, the Greeks, and the Romans have used various treatment baths. In Sparta, hydrotherapy became compulsory: a law was passed requiring every citizen to take a cold bath frequently. Generally, baths used for treatments were either heating baths or cooling baths. Perhaps the Romans developed the bath to the greatest degree. A census in 33 B.C. shows 170 small baths in the city of Rome. 400 years later ~367 A.D. the number increased to 856.

Nearly 1000 years before the Christian era, a debate raged among the Greeks and Romans about the ideals of education and the benefits of physical fitness. Some thought that education should be strictly academic, while other great and influential thinkers, such as Aristotle and Socrates, believed that physical training belongs to liberal arts and music.

In the first century B.C. in Rome many new facilities were being built just for bathing and exercise incorporating new thermal technologies, such as different materials for making cauldrons in which the water was heated and various methods of heating the water (wood, coal, dried manure). Hot baths and exercise were becoming a part of daily life.

The Baths of Caracalla (Rome cir. 212) featured facilities to accommodate 3000 bathers, a swimming pool, parks, sporting area, and an extensive library. Roman baths were very similar to the Greek gymnasiums. The Greek bath "the thermae", had libraries, lecture rooms, and promenades. Masterpiece Statuaries of Greek gods adorned the hallways and promontory. The Roman baths had been very popular for more than six hundred years, but it was during the last century B.C. that their popularity rose to a social institution attended daily—"you were nobody if you weren't at the Roman bathhouse."

In Greek baths, one would bathe and exercise in the nude, but Romans wore tunics suitable for exercise and bathing
Celsus: recommended a light sweat!
Galen: prescribed that all exercise should be followed by massage and sometimes by hot bathing.
The actual bathing proceeded through a series of tubs or pools, always shallow, of increasingly hot water. The final plunge, called the frigidarium, was into cold water.

The Hadrianic Baths at Leptis Magma (126 A.D.) the largest Roman bath was an extensive building complex for entertainment or lectures where one would lounge after exercise, steam bath, or soothing oil massage. The thermae of Rome also offered food and beverages. But not everyone welcomed the thermae's grand architecture, decadent slave girls, food, wine, and general excess. Christians later reflected upon the decadence of Roman baths as evidence of the moral collapse of Roman Society.

The Christian era marks the beginning of the Middle Ages, when medicine, exercise, and all therapeutic measures fell into disuse, and their associated institutions into disarray. The Olympic games were terminated in 393 A.D. ending an era of importance for massage and exercise. Even hygiene fell from its position as centerpiece of the Greco—Roman Health Care. "Medicine" and its literature declined, as did medical gymnastic and massage returning it to its former level or folk medicine. There is virtually no mentioning of massage in the medical literature for centuries after the fall of Rome; it was too "common" to qualify for therapeutic purposes. With the unfold of the Middle Ages the Arab countries, India, China, and several places in Europe have kept the spirit of massage- & Hydrotherapy very much alive.

However in a climate of such negativity toward the body, where all forms of public exhibition as gymnastics was considered un-Christian and everything related to exercise or bath was banned, it was the church that helped preserve massage within the Western world during the Middle Ages. A new home was found within the emerging Christian environment as part of Christian rituals and in the care of the sick and dying.

Numerous attempts were made to restore the deteriorated baths into their former places of learning, culture, and healing. King Charlemagne (742-814), Emperor of the West crowned in 800 A.D. by the Pope, led the revival of many declining baths in his realm, known today as France, Germany, and northern Italy. Other baths were maintained by religious sects like the Benedictine monks who founded the Spa at Bad Ragaz in Switzerland in 740 A. D. The French order of Capuchin built convents at nearly all spas in France. At that time, nuns, priests, and physicians could receive special permission to visit these spas for healing treatments. This way the old spas were used for housing of the religious orders and as healing facilities.

With the Renaissance Period, the medical thinkers of the time looked back to the ancients but also moved forward in a new understanding of anatomical and physiological ways of medical science. By the 16th century a volume of written work on "Mechanical Treatments" was documented from a variety of European countries, including France, Germany, England, and Italy.

Paracelsus (1493-1541) was a medical doctor, alchemist and philosopher, who also was a firm believer of hot and cold springs and the medicinal value of bathing. In 1535 he visited the Spa at Bad Ragaz in Switzerland and wrote a study of its hydrology. He also believed in massage because of its valuable effect on the blood circulation. Paracelsus was also credited for recognizing the value of keeping wounds clean to avoid infection.

Throughout human history, water has been essential for health and spiritual well being as part of ceremonial practices in many religions. The early Egyptians worshiped the Nile; priests were required to bathe in the river twice daily before entering the sacred temples. In India, bathing in the Ganges River is part of the ritual purification. The Talmud teaches the importance of water in personal hygiene and Jewish women have long used the mikvah (a ritual cleansing bath) after menstruation. The first Christian baptism took place in the sacred waters of the Jordan River. Muslims are required to wash the face, hands, and neck in a ritual manner five times a day before each of their daily prayers.

Even though humans live on dry land, our bodies contain more than 60% water by weight creating an aquatic environment. Every single body cell is made of water-rich intracellular fluid and is surrounded by a protective layer of extra-cellular fluid also made primarily of water. The water content is constantly changing by eliminating waste products and replenishing the loss by consuming drinks and fruits. Fluids and minerals can also be absorbed in small amounts via the skin by soaking or bathing in warm water.

Bathing for Health & Healing

Many ancient developments were established near springs and the water was often revered, whether the water contained sulfur, was carbonated, or plain. Most natural springs were eventually developed into baths and then into spas. The first medical study of hot springs in Japan was documented in 1709 and approximately six universities had established medical research institutes at hot springs to evaluate their therapeutic benefits on an ongoing basis. Around 1865, hot spring facilities were being developed in the western United States in cities as well as in remote areas. The spas of Europe during this time were mostly rebuilt upon the ruins of ancient facilities. Whereas new American hot spring resorts were modeled after famous European spas. The two oldest northern California developments still in existence are Wilbur Hot Springs and Harbin Hot Springs. Most spas and hot springs advertised the healing qualities of their waters, usually endorsed by a physician.

Around 1850, water cure establishments started to offer group bathing, hot and cold sheet and blanket wraps, personal sitz baths—along with claims that hydrotherapy could cure everything from heart disease to cancer. The government later prohibited such health claims. Despite that, "modern" naturopathic physicians adopted many hydrotherapy practices and recommended hot or cold bath for many ailments. During the mid 1800's Sebastian Kneipp (1827-1897) developed kneippism—(holistic medicine emphasizing hydrotherapy). Father Kneipp applied his water cure for decades and established the "Central Kneipp Association" in 1890 making his hydrotherapy famous worldwide. Meanwhile, most of America's European—style luxury health spas fell from fashion around World War I (1914-1918) and started slowly to resurrect in the 1970's as relaxation retreats.

Few are aware that balneology has been an integrative part of mainstream medicine in Europe and Japan, where an abundance of scientific documentation is evidence for the medicinal value of physiotherapy if applied appropriately.

"Physiotherapy is the practice of natural therapeutics and treats the body and its abnormalities by natural or physical measures of healing according to the laws of physics and mechanics . More explicitly expressed, it embodies the use of light, heat, water, manipulations, and electricity for their therapeutic effects."

—H. William Baum, Ph.T
NY, NY Jan 1944

According to the physical laws that "Actio causes Reactio" the physiotherapist is trained to calculate the physiological aftereffect of applied therapy. It is not important what you do, it is how you do it, and most important how the patient feels at the end.

Nature Cure

Hydrotherapy used to be a respected treatment method in the United States. Dr. Guy Hinsdale stated in a paper of the American Medical Association in May 1927 that:
"Water may act as powerful stimulus according to its temperature." The Battle Creek Sanitarium developed hydrotherapy to its greatest degree in modern times. Originally founded in 1866 as Western Health Reform Institute, by Adventist church leader Ellen White. The institute provided treatment far ahead of its time with hydrotherapy, rest, sunshine, and controlled diet. Around May 1880, Doctor John Harvey Kellog accepted Ellen White's offer to become the first medical director of the Battle Creek Sanitarium after returning from Europe where he had studied natural healing methods. Dr. Kellog was not only known to be generous to those being unable to pay, he was well created a nutritional program for malnourished children and their mothers in the community. On the other hand, Dr. Kellog also wanted to attract famous and wealthy patrons like Henry Ford, John D. Rockefeller, and Harvey Firestone. During his sixty-seven years as medical director of Battle Creek he was able to introduce innovations in the fields of diet, exercise, hygiene, hydrotherapy, light therapy, and massage.

The training for these modalities used at the Sanitarium was offered in Dr. Kellog's own courses. The official training school for nurses was established in 1883. "The Sanitarium nurse must not only understand the dressing of wound and the general care of sick people, but *must* be skilled in massage and thoroughly familiar with all the principles and methods of hydrotherapy. The facility flourished until the depression began taking away most wealthy clients. The Battle Creek Sanitarium closed in 1938. Dr. Kellog lived until 1942 to the age of 91.

Nature Cure was a system for treating diseases with natural agents such as water, air, diet, and sunshine, which developed in the nineteenth-century in Europe. Not surprisingly, the only significant documentations about the history of nature cure were published in German and have never been translated into English.

Naturopathy was the combination of nature cure and homeopathy, spinal manipulation, and other natural therapies, which were developed in the early 20th century in America.

Naturopathic Medicine is the application of the principles of naturopathy within the context of modern scientific knowledge evolving since the second half of the 20th century. The term nature doctor has been used for practitioners from all three of these permutations of nature-oriented medicine.

There have been numerous excellent practitioners, pioneers in the field of natural remedies who respectfully deserve their place among nature doctors and I truly apologize for not being able to mention them all but it would drift me far away from my original subject—Hydrotherapy—and my intention to explain: "Why what happened When" without neglect nor praise.

Hippocrates (460-377 B.C) "father of medicine" being included in the list of nature doctors may result from his *"vis medicatrix naturae"* or "healing power of nature" which became the basic tenet of the Hippocratic School and remains one of the central themes of naturopathic philosophy.

The Corpus Hippocraticum, the collection of Hippocratic writings, was the work of different authors belonging to two different schools, which symbolized the eternal polarity of medicine. *The School of Cos* represented the vitalistic, empirical approach to health, while *The School of Cnidos* promoted the rationalistic, analytical approach.

Focusing primarily on the vitalistic teachings of Cos, naturopathy is indebted to Hippocrates for formulating its fundamental credo of the *"vis medicatrix naturae"*, which the physician can support but never replace. Hippocrates also realized that treating a disease meant treating the patient as whole.

The word physician (Greek: nature) was used by Hippocrates to denote that every practitioner of medicine was to be skilled in nature and must strive to know what man is in relation to food, drink, occupation, and what effect these have on him. The physician should never forget that disturbances in any organ correspond to a disturbance of the whole person and in order to heal even an eye, one must heal the head and even the whole body.

Paracelsus (1493-1541) besides his praises that "Nature is the physician not man" and "that she will heal all wounds by herself if you prevent infection" did *not* make him part of the Nature Doctors.

Paracelsus's real name was Theophrastus but he defiantly adopted the penname Paracelsus which meant "better than Celsus" the great Roman encyclopedist, who had ruled medical science for centuries. However, Paracelsus, introduced such chemical drugs as antimonial and arsenical compounds, lead nitrates, chlorides of iron and gold, copper, sulphates, bismuth as well as tin compounds. "It was the exaggerated use of such drugs in the medical practice of the early nineteenth century which was one if the main reasons for the "Nature Doctors" to condemn scientific medicine of their times as "poison medicine" and lean away from it.

Unlike Hippocrates or Paracelsus, Christoph Wilhelm Hufeland (1762-1836) was never mentioned as a predecessor in American naturopathic literature. Whereas in Germany he is still honored as example of a truly holistic physician and every year professional organizations of natural therapies award one outstanding member with the Hufeland Medal as recognition.

Hufeland's special concern for public health led him to build the first morgue in Germany to prevent people for being mistakenly buried alive. And in order to contain smallpox, he insisted to quarantine patients. Being a great supporter of watercure and mineral springs which he often prescribed in his own practice, he knew most of the springs in Germany from visiting them, back when he was writing his treatise on mineral springs. His greatest success was his book "*The Art of Prolonging Human Life*, first published in 1796. This became the most widely read book on the subject of preventative medicine. It was reprinted numerous times and translated into many languages, even Chinese. Only Kneipp's *My Water Cure* written a century later had comparable success. Later editions of Hufeland's books were titled: Macrobiotic: The Art of Prolonging Life. Hufeland coined the term "macrobiotics" to describe the art of prolonging life. This term was later borrowed by George Oshawa, who started the modern macrobiotic movement. He was one of Hufeland's greatest admirers. For Hufeland, macrobiotic was different from medical art, he wrote:

> "*The object of the medical art is health; that of macrobiotic, long life...the medical art must consider every disease as an evil, which cannot be too soon expelled; the macrobiotic, on the other hand, shows that many diseases may be the means of prolonging life*"

Hufeland spoke about the curative powers of fever, inflammation and suppuration and how their suppression can cause disease. Most of the basic concepts of later nature doctors can be found in macrobiotic. On the influence of light, he wrote:

> "*Let a plant or an animal be deprived of light, not with standing any nourishment, care, and cultivation, it will first lose its color, than its strength, and at last, entirely decay.*" "*All the melancholy consequences of a sedentary life and overstraining the mental faculties would disappear, if people, some hours every day, or a few months in the year, would take hold of a spade or a mattock and cultivate their field or garden.*"

Hufeland was deeply influenced by the philosopher Jean-Jacques Rousseau (1712-1778) with his call "Return to Nature!" Rousseau must be considered the true spiritual father of the nature cure movement. He regarded medicine as "art more pernicious to men than all the ill it claims to cure." (1979) With his "naturism" Rousseau supplied the ideological basis for nature cure, he provided the nature cure movement with a philosophical foundation.

The three essential elements characterizing nature cure:

1.) A strong emotional attitude towards nature which can be defined as "naturism"

2.) A theory of health, disease, treatment, and cure, which we know as nature cure or naturopathy.

3.) A preference for certain treatment methods, which are considered natural (physiotherapy) such as the application of water, light, air, movement, and diet. (Rothschuh 1983)

One of the most important and influential people in regards of nature cure was J.H Rausse (1805-1848). Born in Guestrow/Mecklenburg (Germany) under the name Heinrich F. Francke. His fellow university students gave him the nickname "Rausse" French term for the German word "Ross" meaning "horse" in respect of his strength and wild temperament.

Rausse was highly influenced by Jean Jacque Rousseau's "Return to Nature" inspiring his idea of living a dissolute life becoming a complete man of nature. He devoted himself entirely to the observation of nature, studied the plants, trees, the origins of springs, rivers, and the formation of weather patterns as well as the behavior of animals. After deciding to live among the Osage Indians in North America as hunter he fell ill with yellow fever and after almost a year he decided to return to Germany to die in his homeland. However the sea journey back to Europe had such a beneficial effect on his health that he regained sufficient strength to continue working as a forester. In addition, he started his career as a writer. The change in his life which later brought him the title as "The Reformer of Water Cure" occurred after his illness flared up again. Due to his aversion to "regular medical treatments" he wrote once concerning medicine: *"I regarded this science as a mindless repetition of an ancient system which had nothing to do with true healing."*
and now he decided to seek help in Priessnitz' Water Cure in 1837, when he spent ten weeks in Graefenberg. He was so profoundly impressed by this completely new approach to healing, its simplicity and closeness to nature that he began to ponder the principles underlying water cure, which Priessnitz followed by intuition. Once discerning the physiological basis of the water cure, he was able to identify errors in its application in certain cases, including his own which prompted his reform of water cure. Rausse wrote: "I returned home after I was clear about the design of my cure" "However, I would have never attained an understanding of the general as well as of my own water cure if Priessnitz' great and ingenious discoveries had not become the basis for my successive research and discoveries." (Cited by Kapp 1850) About his observations in Graefenberg, Rausse wrote a book titled *"The Spirit of the Graefenberg Water Cure"* (1838) which then was sensational. A year later, he published *"Miscellanies to the Graefenberg Water Cure"*, which was dedicated to Priessnitz with the motto "Water can do it" This was the main contribution to Priessnitz fame and recognition. Rausse considered Priessnitz the discoverer of the water cure, but looked at himself as its master and perfecter. Originally, Rausse did not intend to become a "water doctor", but he was pushed into this new career by his enthusiastic readers and admirers. As well was he drawn by the challenge to enter this field professionally because of mistakes in water cure practices, which he felt corrupted the true principles of hydrotherapy. Despite his busy water cure practice in Stuer/Mecklenburg, he still found time to write inflammatory polemics, outstanding in their logic and wit. His last complete work:

Errors of Physicians and others in the Practice of the Water Cure as Remedial Agent in the Prevention and Cure of Medicine. (1847), which condemns the mistakes of physicians who were using water in the "wrong way" or in combination with drugs. By 1847, he moved his Stuer establishment to a larger water-cure institution in Lehsen/Wittenberg and soon in April of 1848 to Alexandersbad/Wunsiedel. Here he began to write the first part of his book, *Instructions for the Use of the Water Cure Methods* (1850), part two and three were completed after his death by his cousin and disciple Theodor Hahn (1824-1883).

Nature Cure and its chronological "stepping stones" creations of terminology.

Jean Jacque Rousseau (1712-1778)
Considered the true spiritual father of the nature cure movement
Vincent Priessnitz (1799-1852)
The discoverer of water cure

J.H. Rausse (1805-1848)
The reformer and perfecter of water cure

Benedict Lust (1872-1925)
The Father of Naturopathy

Henry Lindlahr (1862-1963)
Founder of Scientific Naturopathy

Father Sebastian Kneipp (1824-1897)
Founder of Kneippism (Kneipp Kur)
Refined from Vincent Priessnitz Water Cure
Kneipp also introduced herbalism into nature cure

Adolf Just (1859-1936)
Also inspired by Jean Jacque Rousseau
"Return to Nature" became his main ideal
Discovery of the healing power of earth or geotherapy became his main contribution to nature cure.

Emmanual Felke (1856-1926)
Specifically used clay which brought him the title "The Clay Pastor"

This leads to a closer look at the individual nature doctors, their discoveries and political challenges of their times and their contributions to nature cure. As successful pharmaceutical companies began to financially support medical school's in the U.S., as they offered aid and loans to medical students, and as pharmaceutical manufactures began to serve on the board of directors at medical schools around the country during the first half of the twentieth century, these financial giants changed the curriculum at schools to downplay the importance of water therapy and herbs while emphasizing drugs to kill disease or surgery to remove the disease. This unfortunate change in teaching methods stressed technology in America, whereas the use of hydrotherapy, mineral springs, and herbal remedies remained constant throughout the European continent. The main difference was that in Europe, doctors embraced both the past of medicine and technological advances from America. However American doctors abandoned time-tested methods of hydrotherapy preferring drugs and surgeries. As a result, we are seeing resurgence in popularity with more natural methods of healing in America, as people become dissatisfied with modern medical industry.

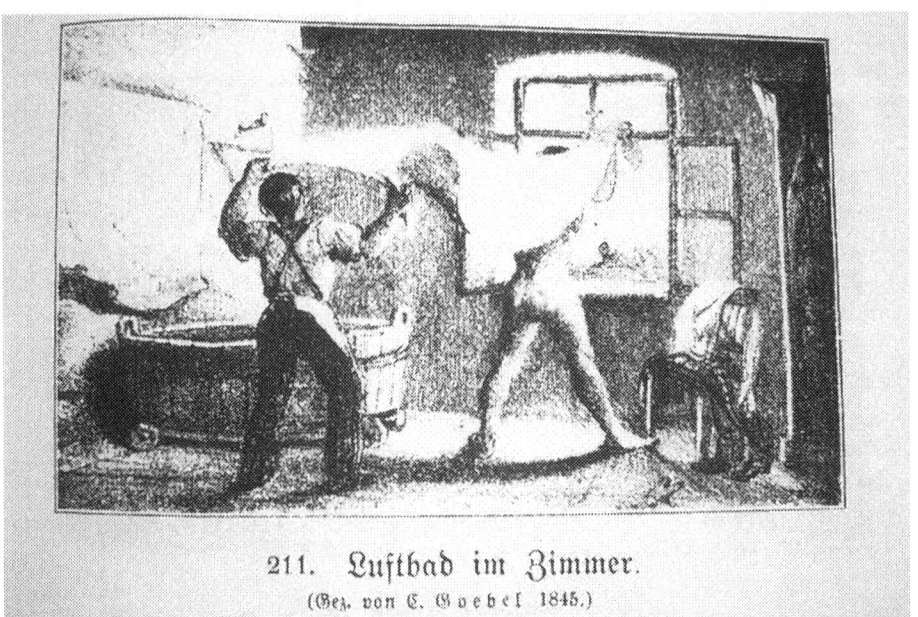

211. Luftbad im Zimmer.
(Gez. von C. Goebel 1845.)

Airbath indoors

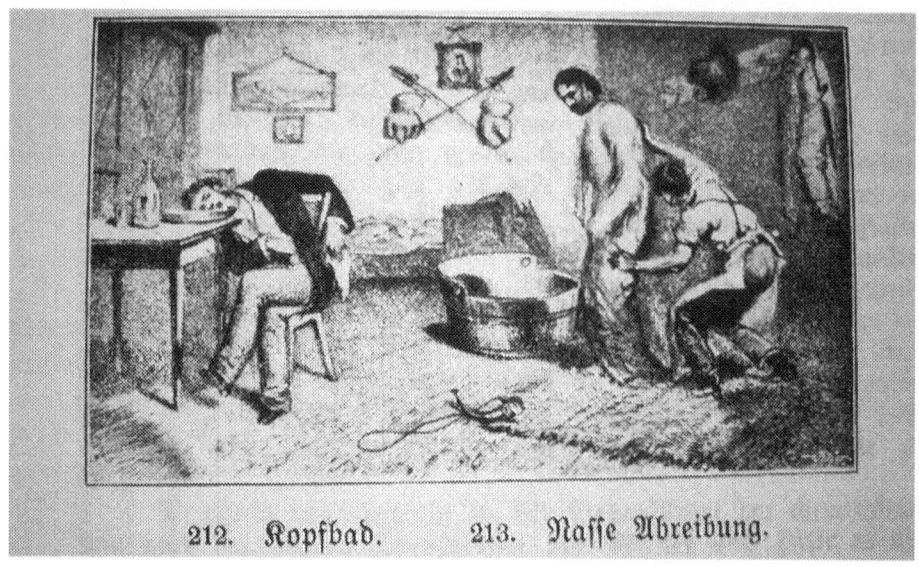

212. Ropfbad.   213. Naffe Abreibung.

Headbath & Wet towel bath (friction)

Nature Doctors and their integrative approach to therapy from the 18th to the 20th century.

Many of our famous nature doctor pioneers were, whether philosophically inspired by writings or challenged by their own failing health, desperate to find help or possible cure, leading to refining and improving therapies. With growing technology and physiological understanding even interest of scientific explanation led to the combination of remedies moving those to a higher level of sophistication.

1. Foundations of Nature Cure

Vincent Priessnitz (1799-1852) became one of the most famous healers of the 19th century, despite the fact that he never went to medical school. He enabled the establishment of hydrotherapy to become a legitimate medical entity, which allowed those simple methods of natural healing of his time to revolve into naturopathic medicine of today.

Priessnitz was born October 4th, 1799 in Graefenberg close to the village of the early water doctors Sigmund Hahn (1664-1773). The Hahn's used cold water therapies extensively in their medical practice. When Priessnitz had to quit school to take care of the family farm as a fairly young boy, an old man in the neighborhood supposingly showed him how to treat injured cattle with water. Shortly after, Priessnitz was credited with curing his father's feverish cow by cold-water application. While working in his father's mountain pasture he was watching a wounded stag hobble into a mountain spring and situate itself with the injured limb submerged in the cold flowing water. The stag returned each day to treat itself and improved day by day until it finally got well. Working on the farm Priessnitz experienced a number of injuries giving him the opportunity to practice the healing powers of cold water on himself. When he was thirteen he sprained his wrist and he noticed that it felt much better under the cold stream of a water pump. Since he could not keep his wrist under the pump he wrapped it in a wet bandage while taking care of his chores. The "Priessnitz compress" was born! Later it was adopted into regular medical practice and can be still found today in medical dictionaries. When he was seventeen, Priessnitz got run over by a horse-drawn wagon carrying wood. The local surgeon considered the critical injuries incurable, but Priessnitz set his own broken ribs by himself by pressing his abdomen against the edge of an armchair and bound himself with a bandage wrung out in cold water. He moistened the bandage whenever it was dry and drank large amounts of cold water. After ten days, he was up again attending to his chores. For the following years, he wore the bandage as support after which he pronounced himself fully recovered. Now he felt obligated to share his discoveries with others; and whenever he heard of anyone being injured, he recommended cold-water treatments as he had applied to himself. Applying sponge ablutions, he soon was known as "Schwamm" or "Sponge-doctor" In the beginning he did not charge for his services and made numerous house calls, but he learned from experience that people who came to him and paid for treatment were cured most quickly. Benedict Lust stated in 1918; "Even in Priessnitz days, there was already a jealous medical profession." Since Priessnitz's success diminished regular doctors practices, he was frequently arrested and tried for illegal practice of medicine; but he was always acquitted because he used only water, not medicine. These persecutions did not embitter Priessnitz; he accepted them with equanimity and silence since they rather spread his fame attracting more patients. One physician sent by the state to investigate Priessnitz thereafter frequently referred patients to Graefenberg. At one point, in frustration, authorities had raided Priessnitz's place and wrecked it in search of his secret "drug". They cut up all his sponges but the mystery was not revealed. In 1829 the magistrate prohibited him from using his "bewitched "sponges. Priessnitz' s reply: "This is even better; then I use only my hands: "Thus life comes to life!" And from then on Priessnitz never used sponges again only the flat hand for applying water, which he noticed, was even more effective.

Long before Priessnitz, the value of cold water was known by the Hahn's, for instance, and the great water cure propagandist, Eucharius Ferdinand Christian Oertel (1765-1850); but they had not really understood its many possibilities. In his Priessnitz book Philo vom Walde listed fifty-six different cold-water applications. Besides members of the royalty and clerical dignitaries Chopin, Gogol, and Napoleon III have been among his patients. With growing success, complaints against Priessnitz from the medical profession escalated proportionately. In 1838, the Austrian government created a special commission to investigate Priessnitz. Baron Turkheim, head of this commission, traveled to Graefenberg to settle this matter. Turkheim's report to the Imperial Cabinet at Vienna is worth quoting in full length.

> "That Priessnitz is no ordinary man even his enemies must admit. He is no imposter, but is filled with the purest zeal to help others whenever he is asked to do so; and he is particularly fitted to do this. The number of those, who call Priessnitz a quack and a man of selfish motives, only constitute a small minority, and are mostly doctors and surgeons from the surrounding districts whose incomes are reduced by his practice, and who therefore get up complaints against him. Unassuming, modest, ever ready to give his patients help, untiring by day and night, obliging, firm and consistent in his actions, Priessnitz possesses qualities, which are inadmissible in an imposter. Not withstanding the most careful investigations, I have been unable to trace a single instance wherein he was activated by selfish motives."

After this stunning endorsement the Austrian government decreed that Priessnitz should enjoy the same privileges as medical doctors, and that no one should ever harass him again. The government even built new roads to facilitate access to Priessnitz's institute. When finally the Emperor of Austria honored Priessnitz with a large gold medal for civic merit, the highest mark of distinction in Austria, the almost two decades of prosecution and harassment ended and Priessnitz was allowed to practice healing as he saw fit.

Priessnitz could read, but his writing skills were limited. His only book, "*Familien—Wasserbuch*" (Family Water book), was sketchy. In order to learn his therapeutic approach, interested physicians had to travel to Graefenberg to observe, which they did in large numbers. In 1839, one hundred twenty doctors came to study from Priessnitz, his students had to follow close by his side and observe for weeks at a time. Only through their writings and notes, records of the Priessnitz methods were kept. Priessnitz preferred soft water over mineral water because of its ability to dissolve impurities. He never used hot water because he thought it was debilitating. Priessnitz had a general pattern of therapy but no two patients were treated alike. He was a genius in the art of individual treatment (Detmar 1951). He rejected all rule-of-thumb therapy "Our task is not to treat disease, but the patient". *He individualized his treatments according to his own system of diagnosis based on close observation of the patient and the reaction of the skin to cold-water treatment, which he often timed with a watch.* A complete cure could take from four weeks up to two years. Priessnitz also treasured the value of fresh air, he was an absolute air fanatic, which was fundamental for the development of the air bath of the later back-to-nature movement. The windows in his sickrooms had to stand open all the time. One of his statements quoted by Schoenberger 1931 was : "If I had no water, I could cure with air!" Air was used as a thermal and as a mechanical stimulant. In his "air-water bath" patients did not dry with towels but had to create a draft by beating the wet body with a sheet to activate inactive skin. His idea was that people should warm themselves by exercise and not heavy clothes. In fact, Priessnitz considered heat from external sources a bad thing not only in water and clothing but also in food. It is known that Priessnitz treated over 40,000 patients, thousands of people came from all over the world, including Peru, Egypt, Brazil, even Lapland. Graefenberg was a remote location in an age of difficult transportation, 260 miles from Berlin, 200 miles from Dresden, and 175 miles from Vienna. Back then it took 10-14 days to get to Graefenberg from England via steamboat, railway, and carriage.

Despite his busy practice he was a devoted family man. When he married his wife in 1828, she did not have too much faith in Priessnitz therapies and she insisted that their children be treated by orthodox doctors to which Priessnitz agreed. However, when one of the children contracted measles and died under the regular doctors care, she started to believe that her husband's therapeutic approaches where right. From that time on she never had any doubts and even adopted the water treatment for her own health.

Priessnitz was a careful observer; a good judge of human nature, and his mechanical skills enabled him to invent various technical modifications of water treatment.

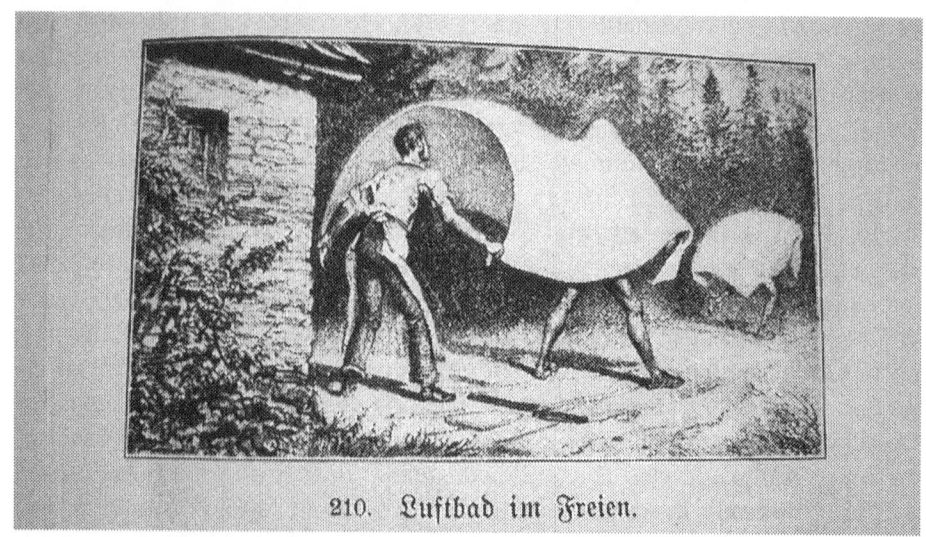

210. Luftbad im Freien.

Airbath outdoors

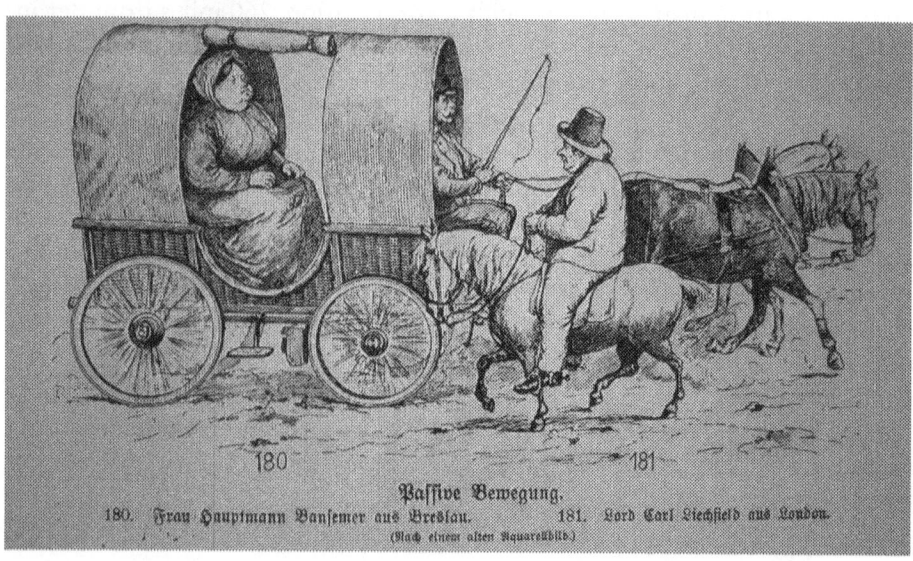

Passive Bewegung.
180. Frau Hauptmann Bansemer aus Breslau.   181. Lord Carl Liechfield aus London.
(Nach einem alten Aquarellbild.)

Passive Exercise

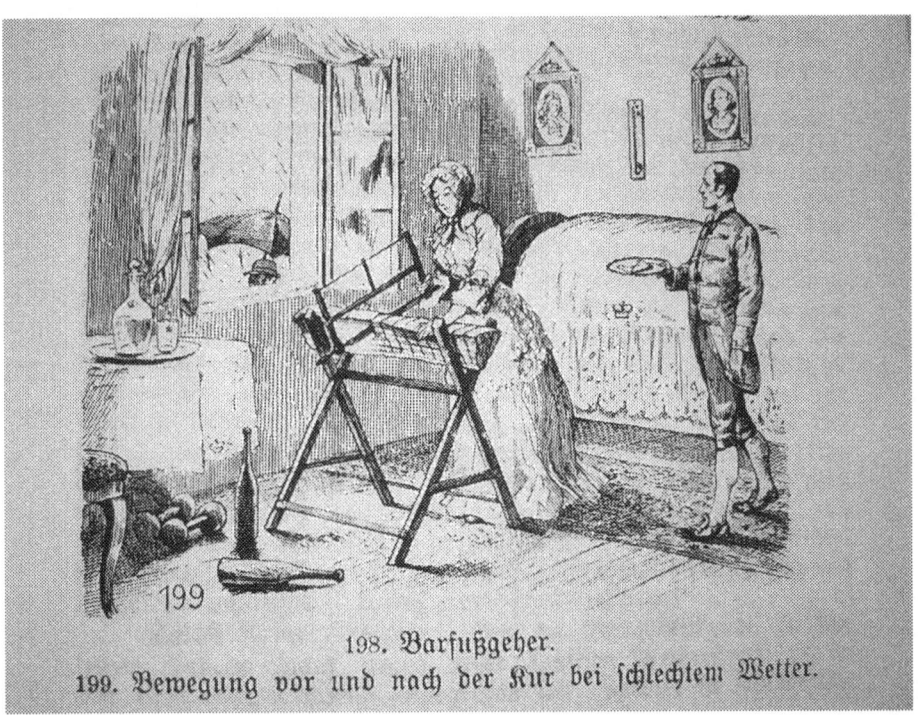

198. Barfußgeher.
199. Bewegung vor und nach der Kur bei schlechtem Wetter.

Exercise indoors during bad weather

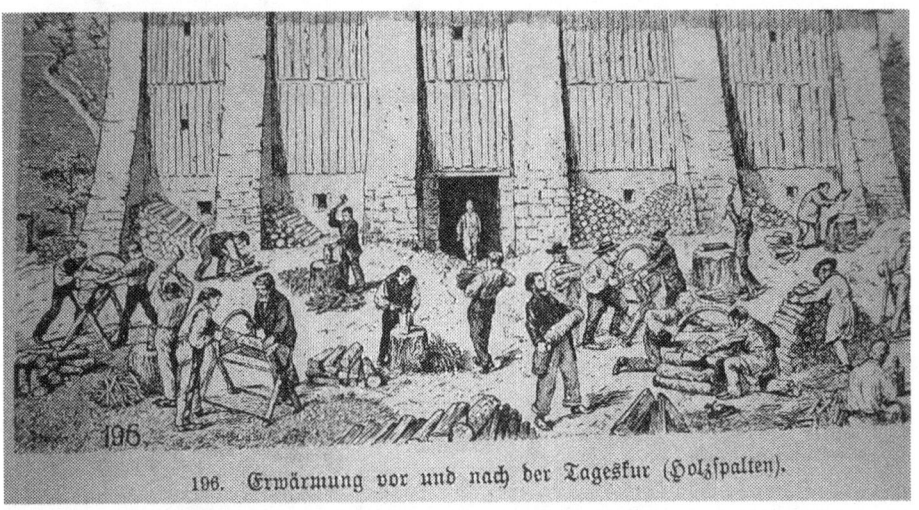

196. Erwärmung vor und nach der Tageskur (Holzspalten).

Warming up before and after treatments

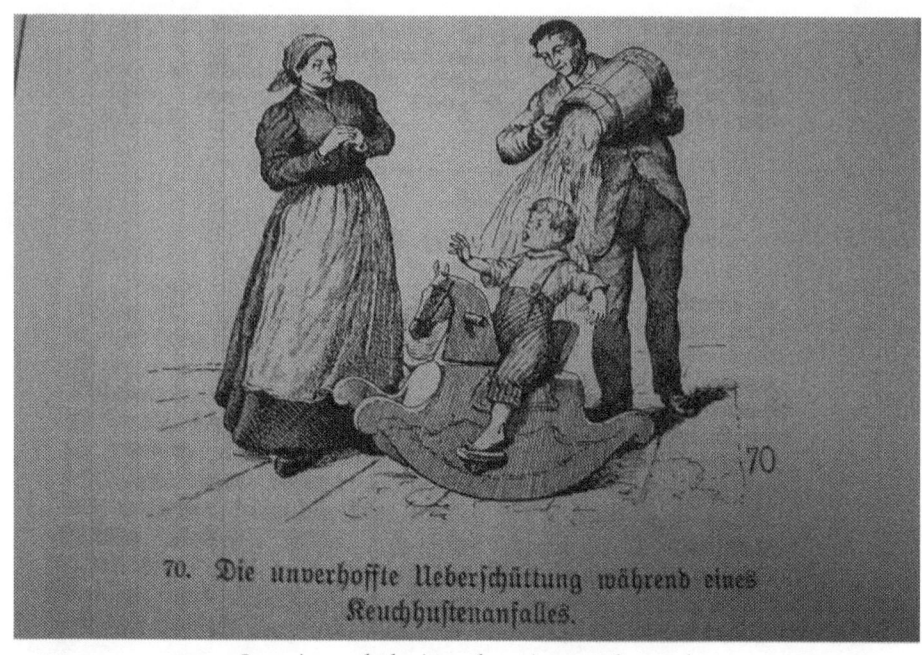

70. Die unverhoffte Ueberschüttung während eines
Keuchhustenanfalles.

Surprise gush during whopping cough attack

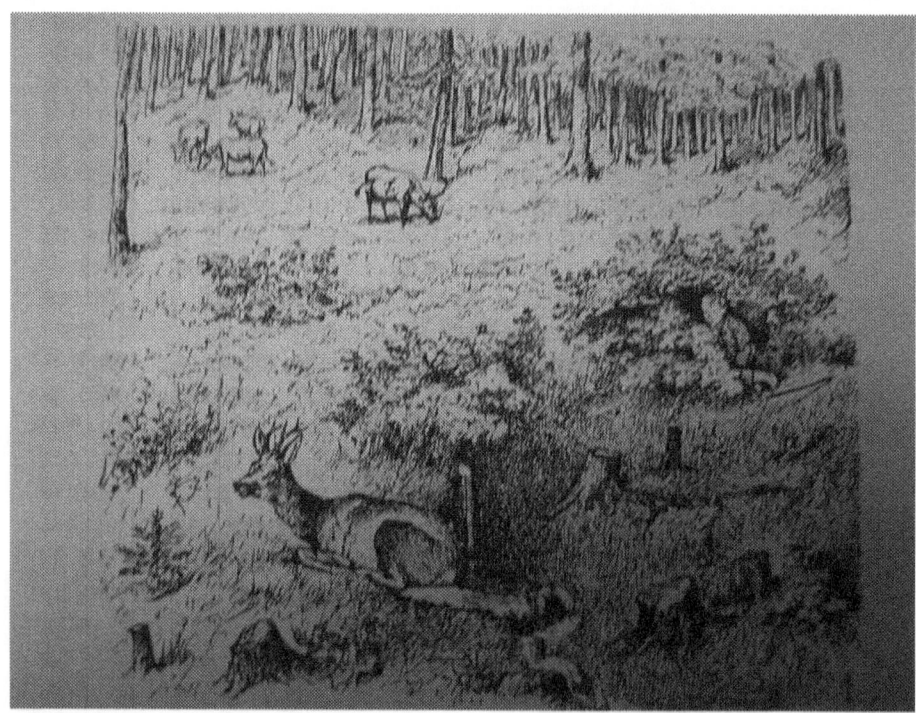

Despite his lack of scientific training Priessnitz became an amazingly success-ful doctor. He rejected the offer to access medical literature saying he was afraid they would warp his mind. "Doctors have learned too much," he used to say, "If they want to be good water doctors, they would have to forget a lot."

Priessnitz has always been granted the status as "Father of Hydrotherapy" but was rarely acknowledged as the progenitor of naturopathic medicine. His importance to the history of naturopathic medicine arose from being the first person to whom the term "Naturarzt" (nature doctor) was given as well as being the first to systematize and promote a natural method of healing which was comprised "externally of pure water, fresh air, skin friction, kneading, and light clothing; internally of simple diet, pure water drinking in conjunction with open air exercise." He also believed in toxicity as a basis of disease, the idea of chronic disease as a result of suppressive treatments of acute disease.

Upon request of his family, after Priessnitz's death, Josef Schindler, M.D. (1814-1891) continued the methods of his teacher in exemplary fashion in Graefenberg for nearly forty years. Schindler introduced hydrotherapy to Wilhelm Winternitz (1834-1912), a professor from the University of Vienna, who established a scientific basis for it and taught it to Simon Baruch (1840-1921) and John Harvey Kellog (1852-1943). These American medical doctors brought Priessnitz methods successfully to the United States.

Priessnitz success in a nutshell, stemmed from removing patients from their stress-ful environment that often induced their illness and placing them into a pleasant communal setting, implementing diet and exercise which strengthened the body, he had paved the way for Kneipp, Lust, Lindlahr, and all future Nature Doctors by popularizing treatments throughout the western world.

2.) Priessnitz Rival: Moist Heat, Thirst, and Fasting Cure

Johann Schroth (1798-1856) was the total antagonist to Priessnitz' therapeutic approach, he was against cold water applications and prescribed long-lasting warm moist packs, warm water bottles, and hot baths. He prohibited drinking cold-water but he allowed his patients to drink a few glasses of warm wine. His patients were ordered to rest and only move around in moderation and his dietary recommendations were basically salt and fat-free, no meat or milk. Fasting was rediscovered as supplement to the water cure.

Schroth was born in Lindewiese where he grew up and later opened his insti-tute. Lindewiese was a picturesque river valley at the foot of Graefenberg, not far from Priessnitz. Both went to school in Freiwaldau and like Priessnitz, Schroth started to work on the family farm at an early age also observing nature and animals.

Schroth and his cure never reached the same proportions as the Priessnitz water cure. By 1836 when Priessnitz was already famous, Schroth was still unknown. Even though he never claimed that his method was a universal remedy, he endured the same share of persecutions and humiliations. He was accused of being a sorcerer and a quack, persecuted and even thrown into jail. Ultimately in 1840, Schroth was granted official permission to operate his establishment by the authorities that had previously granted Priessnitz the freedom to practice; like Priessnitz, Schroth did not leave any written documentations of his method. However, numerous books and articles about the Schroth cure were published by his successors. Up to today the Schroth cure is still alive and practiced like the Kneipp cure in Germany. Lindewiese belongs now to the Czech Republic and lost its significance after World War II when the Germans were forced to leave. Dr. Herman Brosig saved the Schroth cure by bringing it over to then West Germany in 1949, where it remained in Oberstaufen, the Bavarian Alps, until today. "Lipova Lazne" the old Lindewiese became a tiny spa offering treatment for obesity and rheumatism.

Despite the early translation of Clemens Gehrkes 's book into English about the Schroth cure in children's diseases (1881) and several articles by Dr. Max Mader in the "Naturopath", Schroth's methods never became popular in America. It is speculated that the lack of health spa tradition and certainly the lack of insurance coverage of natural remedies was the main reason. In addition, fast-paced American life is not conductive to take one or even two months for a complete body overhaul. "The Schroth cure requires extraordinary willpower and self-discipline" Schroth's motto was:" Without battle no victory, without deprivation no enjoyment, without cleansing no healing" (Mader 1926) Lust wrote about Priessnitz and Schroth: "Here you have two masters, they are using nature's agents but each one uses it in a different way, and both arrive at the same end". "Their principles constitute basic naturopathy".

3.) The Reformer of Water Cure
J.H Rausse (1805-1848)
Ernest Knapp gave Rausse the title: "Reformer of Water Cure" in his biography written shortly after Rausse's death. Philo vom Walde recognized Rausse as the first man to lay down the scientific principles of hydrotherapy (1898). Richard Metcalfe, the great British hydrotherapist, called Rausse "the most energetic in

propagating the new method of healing in Germany." Rausse's accomplishments have been explained in the previous paragraph "Nature Cure".

4.) Water Cure and Vegetarism

Theodor Hahn (1824-1883), even though he is an important figure in the nature cure movement he is fairly unknown in the United States, because none of his works have been translated into English. Hahn started exclusively with water cure but when he added dietetics and vegetarisim to nature cure, he pushed his influence into the beginning of the health and life reform movement. Hahn's fame was never spread to America like Priessnitz's and Kneipp's. He preserved and extended Rausse's work. Hahn deserves recognition for the important role he played in the development of naturopathic medicine by helping to establish "Nature Cure" as a term and concept. Brauchle wrote in 1951 that Hahn, like so many other nature doctors was inspired by his own sufferings, and disappointments with conventional medicine.

5.) Discovery of the Atmospheric Cure.

Arnold Rikli (1823-1906), little is known about him in America since none of his writings have been translated into English and hardly any literature exists about him in English. His famous saying is quoted occasionally: "Water is good; air is better, but light is the best of all." Rikli was the first who called the attention of the world to the value of light, air, and sunbath. In Germany and Switzerland around the turn of the 20th century nature cure associations competed with each other to establish light and air-baths in many large cities (Heliotherapy). Propagated by the nature cure associations heliotherapy finally gained general recognition with the result that air and sunbathing have become a common activity. Even physicians have not completely forgotten Rikli.

In 1997 the Rikli Award was presented to Prof. Hans Meffert and Dr. H. P. Schorf of the Charite' Humboldt University Berlin for their research on the bio positive systemic effects of optic rays on humans. In 1994, Douglas E. Brash, PhD, associate professor, Dept. of Therapeutic Radiology at Yale School of Medicine was honored with the Rikli Award for his understanding research in Photobiology. The Rikli Award is intended to honor studies that advance the field of photobiology. Arnold Rikli established his first institution for heliotherapy at Veldes, Krain, Austria in 1848, and his sun-treatment has been used in Europe in all drug-less institutions ever since. Heliotherapy has also been taught at the American school of Naturopathy, 7 West 76th Street, NY, NY ever since its establishment in 1896.

6.) The World's Most Famous Nature Doctor

Sebastian Kneipp (1824-1897) a humble priest from an tiny mountain village became one of the most famous people in the world by treating thousands of sick people with natural remedies like pure water, fresh air, exercise, and herbs besides teaching millions about the remedies through his popular health writings. Kneipp like many other natural health pioneers before him started to investigate natural remedies for his own health. After improving his maladies with simple remedies constantly adjusting those till his full recovery, he also felt obligated to help others in his parish. Kneipp's water treatment was originally inspired by Johann Sigmund Hahn's book "Lectures on the Wonderful Healing Power of Fresh Water" which he found in the court library Munich. Too poor to afford professional medical help, Kneipp treated himself with cold water according to this book. Even though the applications were most exceedingly violent and severe he proceeded for six months and at that time noticed no dramatic improvement but he also was encouraged because his disease had not gotten worse. During the winter of 1849 he bathed in the icy water of the Danube two or three times a week for a few minutes. Now he started to notice a small benefit. When Kneipp was ordained as a priest in 1858 he started also to treat his ill parishioners with his already modified cold water system, not so harsh as he had endured. In 1854 he was known as the "Cholera—vicar" because of the many lives he saved with his treatments during an epidemic. In 1855, Kneipp was sent to Woerishofen and immediately founded a school and an orphanage for the poor children. In time the parish flourished, and the fame of Father Kneipp's healing methods spread and he attracted patients from all over the world. Many wealthy people tried to request preferred treatment or having Father Kneipp travel to them, which he reluctantly refused. With one exception, Pope Leo XIII, he was the first and only person Father Kneipp left his parish to treat.

The healing effect of water in conjunction with herbs reflected the universal harmony Kneipp saw in the purpose of God's creation. Father Kneipp's treatment methods were distinguished by individualization and gentleness.

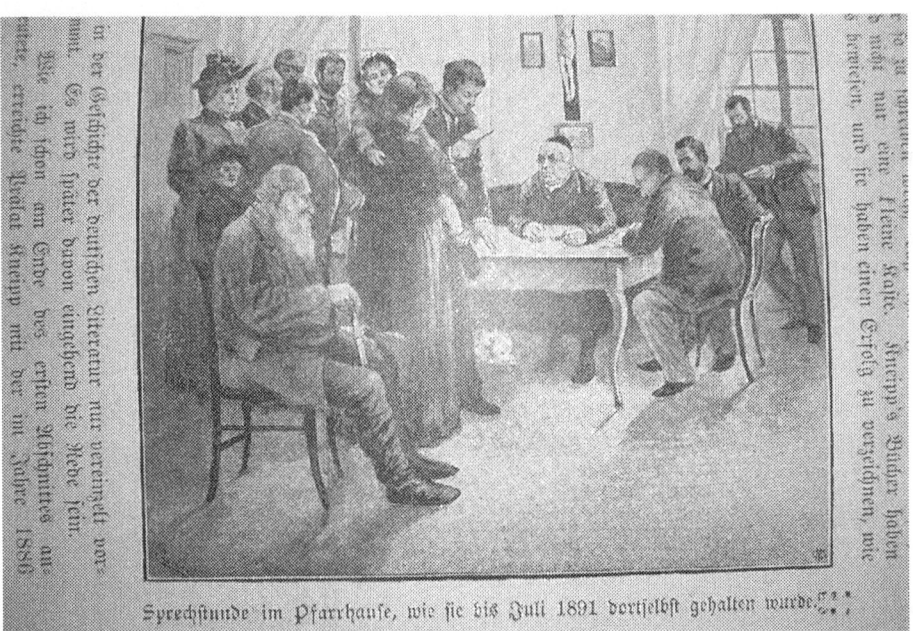

Kneipp is seeing patients in his parish hall until July 1891

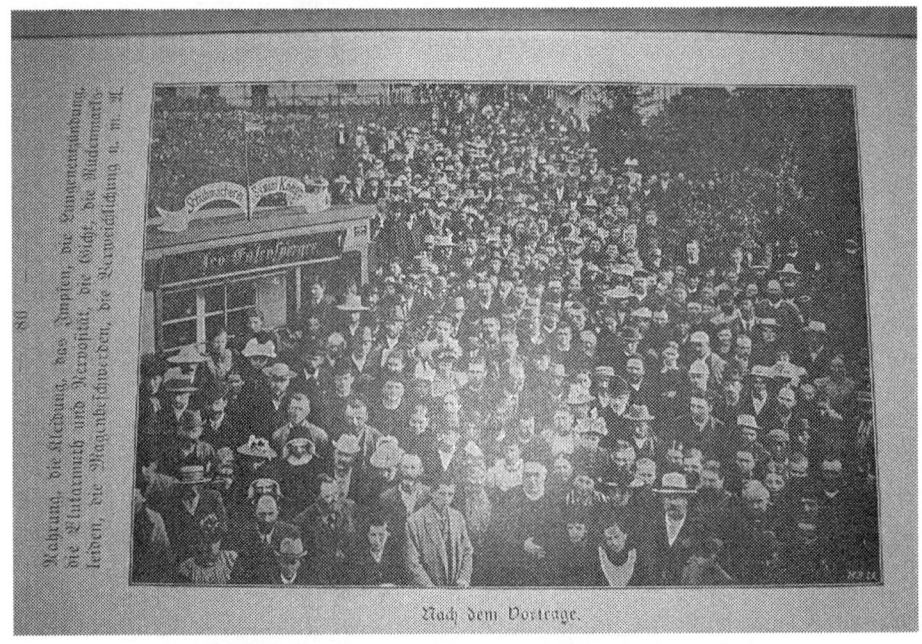

Kneipp and his listeners after his lecture in the park

He wrote in 1893, "*Patients are too often treated in a stereotyped general fashion, and far too little stress is laid on the peculiarities of each separate case,*".

Kneipp utilized wraps, packs, baths, and steaming baths, but his major contribution to hydrotherapy was his discovery of the cold gush or pour. Which is an affusion to a specific part of the body administered from a watering can or unnozzled hose. Each application was very short, often only a minute long and could be timed by his watchless patients by reciting two paternosters. As a healer Kneipp was not rigid, he was always willing to learn from his observations and refine his methods. Kneipp's mother, an experienced herbalist, taught him the use of herbs for various conditions at an early age. So it is no surprise that Kneipp started to experiment with herbal extracts. He became the first to introduce herbalism into nature cure.

Kneipp's most specific influence in America has been on naturopathic medicine. He inspired Benedict Lust and Henry Lindlahr to become naturopaths and establish his healing principles in their country. Prior to that he had cured their life threatening illnesses so they could accomplish their task. The hydropathic movement inspired originally by Priessnitz had prepared the ground, and Kneipp's nature cure combined with Lust's natural therapies brought to a scientific level by Henry Lindlahr developed into naturopathy, which over the course of the twentieth century evolved into naturopathic medicine. The commonly known Kneipp cure in Germany was not widely known or accepted here because America had never developed spa culture like Europe, which provided the right environment for Kneipp's water application. (Kneippism)

7.) The First Big City Nature Doctor
Louis Kuhne (1835-1901) had beside Father Kneipp the greatest influence on Benedict Lust and Henry Lindlahr. Lust was so impressed with Kuhne's two books that he reprinted them, promoted them, and used them as text books in his American School of Naturopathy. Kuhne was the first big city nature doctor; all other so far, Priessnitz, Schroth, Hahn, Kneipp, and Rikli founded their health resorts in the country within beautiful nature settings. Kuhne's establishment was in the city of Leipzig, which created the model for other natural healers to open facilities within large cities where the demand for a more natural life and treatment was the greatest. Henry Lindlahr inspired by Kneipp's example established his sanitarium in Elmhurst, Illinois near Chicago.

Like with many other nature pioneers before him, it was also the inability to find appropriate medical help for his own poor health, which led Louis Kuhne to nature cure. But since all the baths, packs, enemas, and douches gave him only temporary relief he invented a whole new system. On October 1883, he opened the "Louis Kuhne Establishment for the Science of Healing without Medicine and without operation" in Leipzig. Kuhne stated: "My method of curing and new system of diagnosis, the science of facial expressions, proved successful in thousands of cases, and I was able to save many from serious danger by foretelling future illnesses".

In 1894, he published "*The New Science of Healing*" which was almost as popular as Kneipp's "*My Water Cure*". Kuhne praised the early natural applications: "*I have found it necessary, however, to follow more the great discovery and founders of the system—Priessnitz, Schroth, Rausse, and Theodor Hahn—rather than it later representatives. The later, in their excessive zeal for individualization, ran the risk of degenerating into artificially and deviating from the dear and simple path of nature.*"

Kuhne is remembered for his doctrine of the "Unity of Disease" and The Science of Facial Expression but mostly for his friction hipbath and friction sitz bath. Even Gandhi considered those as the most important contribution to hydrotherapy.

8.) *Return to Nature*
Adolf Just (1859-1936) was an enthusiastic follower of Jean—Jacques Rousseau (1712-1778) and his philosophy of naturism. Just shared Rousseau's contempt for civilization and science and indulged in the same romantic idealization of nature. Just's most original contribution to nature cure was the discovery of the healing power of the earth or geotherapy. Besides his love for nature he also had his own health problems and disappointments with orthodox medicine, which brought him to Nature Cure. He wrote in 1903: "In my sufferings I naturally consulted, first, the old school physicians. I called in celebrated doctors and university professors, but they could not help me. In the direst distress and despair I finally lost my high opinion of science. What did I care about science, I wanted help nothing but help."

Just condemned everything that was not in accordance with a natural life: polluting automobiles, closed-in modern housing, deforming styles of clothes and modern chemical agriculture. For every problem, he tried to find a simple natural solution, including funeral procedures. He also rejected warm baths, vapor baths, electric light baths, and massage. Even gymnastics did not meet his approval." I for my part cannot see anything natural in all this artificial bending, winding, straining, stretching, in these gymnastic feats indoors. "(Just 1903) Just elevated the "Luvos Healing Clay" into an almost divine substance and at the same time indignantly condemned the "normal clay". "Luvos Healing Clay" is still available today. (Heilerde-Gesellschaft Luvos Just GmbH & Co., Friedrichsdorf/Germany)

9.) *The Clay or Loam Pastor*
Emanuel Felke (1856-1926) became famous as the "Kneipp of Repelen", a little town where he established his first "Jungborn". Pastor Erdmann Leopold Emmanuel Felke unlike other nature doctors, he joined nature cure because of his interest in natural remedies, his father used simple homeopathic remedies and herbal teas to cure minor illnesses. Felke became famous when he successfully treated members of his congregation during a severe diphtheria epidemic in 1894, because none of the parish's children died after he treated them with the homeopathic remedy, "*Mercuris cyanatus*", unlike children in neighbor villages. Felke did not document his therapies himself, we know about his methods only through his students. Pastor Felke's special gifts as a healer started to attract many desperate patients and soon he was unable to devote himself to his favorite endeavor, the scientific theology. His success treating ailments with homeopathic remedies increased his interest in nature cure and he began to study the treatment methods of Priessnitz, Kneipp, Rikli, Kuhne, and Just, as well as those from Ragnar Berg, Max Bircher—Benner and Heinrich Lahmann. Felke was amazed to be able to detect diseases and their causes in the earliest stages and became a master of facial and iris diagnosis. The originator of iridology was the Hungarian physician and homeopath Ignatz von Peczely (1826-1911), he published his only book,

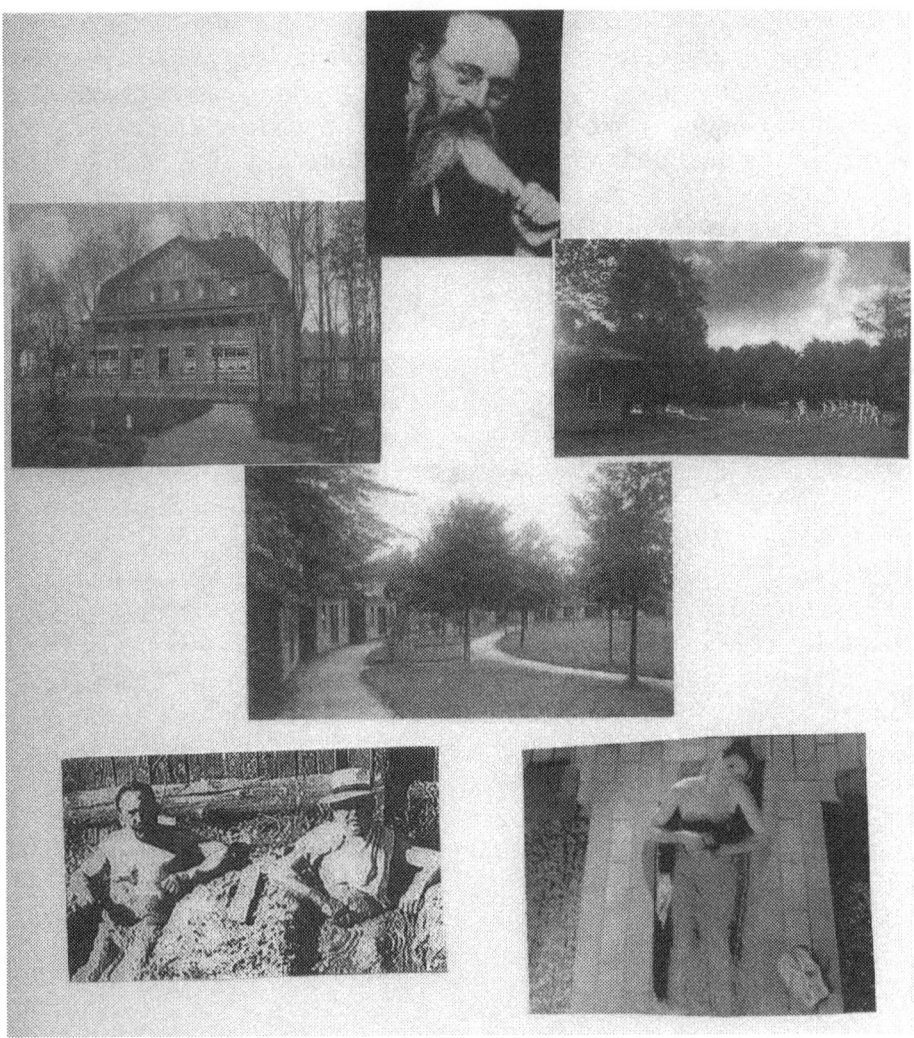

"Discoveries in the Realms of Nature and Art of Healing" in 1873. In 1880, this book was translated into German and was given to Felke by a friend. Benedict Lust credited Felke for his topographical drawing of an iris, "as developing iris diagnosis to the point of almost mathematical exactness". Like Rikli and Just, he envisioned a therapeutic setting close to nature where patients could escape their accustomed environments and enjoy the benefits of light, air, sun, and healthy food. After visiting Just's Jungborn, Felke created the Repelen Jungborn Society LTD. The completed Repelen-Jungborn could house up to 400 patients. The facility had two large light and air parks, one for men and

one for women, surrounded by high wooden fences, where naked patients took light, air, water, and loam baths and engaged in gymnastics twice a day. Inside the two parks were 50 air huts with two to four rooms, to guarantee maximum access to fresh air those had no doors or windows, only curtains for privacy. In the beginning the spa offered friction sitz bath as well as Just's "Earth-and sand-bath" and in 1912 Felke introduced the loam bath, which made him famous as the "Loam Pastor". Felke's view of disease was similar to that of other nature doctors of his time: "Blockages in the eliminative organs—skin, lungs, kidneys, and intestine cause an accumulation of harmful substances." "Every chronic ailment is a disease of the total person, never only of a single organ." Felke is also one of the few nature cure doctors who visited America but refused to stay even after a grateful patient offered to build a hospital and a church for him. Felke's "Loam bath" was a considerable improvement to Just's rather crude "earth bath": For the loam bath, low trenches 120 cm (47 inches) long, 60 cm (23 inches) wide and 40-50 cm (16-20 inches) deep, were filled with fresh loam stirred into a mash with water. At Felke's time patients had to dig their own trenches, today patients are assigned to their own bath for the duration of their stay. The bath is taken 30-45 minutes once or twice a day. Felke's legacy, like Schroth's and Kneipp is still alive in Germany. Medical doctors in Germany basically became the successors of Priessnitz, Schroth, Kneipp, and Felke prescribing Hydro-Balneo-and Medicinal Bath therapy for their patients. Medical doctors now equip nature cure sanitariums with the most modern spa facilities. The national health insurance generally pays for the patients care if the doctor considers it medically necessary. "The Pastor Felke Institute for Iris Diagnosis and Wholistic* Therapy in Heinshein" devotes itself to the training of qualified iridologists on a scientific basis.

* *Because of the fact that the subject of hydrotherapy roots in German documentations, some words may have more than one correct way of spelling, f.i. holistic-wholistic*

10.) *The First Scientific Nature Doctor*

Heinrich Lahmann (1860-1905) even as a student, his main interests were dietetics and disease prevention. Not satisfied with the theories and results of scientific medicine, he deeply explored nature cure literature. Before Lahmann started to take over as head of the nature cure institute in Chemnitz, he toured most of the important nature cure establishments to learn the best therapies available. His mathematical thinking led him to this statement of how to determine the common denominator of therapies, which would yield a rational theory:

"*Each one who practices the nature cure method uses it in a different way: one more complicated, one simpler, one fights a disease with low temperatures which another tries to master with higher temperatures, etc. It is impossible to point to the success of one method, in order to prove its absolute correctness, when the same success is achieved with a different method, if for example, the different methods A,B, and C achieve the same goal, then this is proof that all three contain an unknown quantity X which guarantees that success, and that the rest of the procedure is redundant if not harmful. Our task in the future will be to find this quantity X, only then will we have a theory, only then a rational, scientific nature cure and only then a guarantee for the universal dissemination and continuation of a pure method."* (Lahmann 1886)

Lahmann's scientifically trained mind brought a refreshing breeze of systematic thinking to the field of nature cure, previously chaotic with speculations for the reasons of success of different methods. Despite his relatively short life, he left a rich legacy of publications. In his book, *"The Most Important Chapters of the Natural Healing Method"* he described his use of specific gravity as a simple measure for health assessment. He determined the specific gravity by dividing the body weight by the volume of water displaced. The specific gravity of a healthy person fluctuates between 1065 and 1072. Anything below indicated adipose degeneration. Despite his fame in Germany, in America Lahmann enjoys only name recognition, the details of his work are hardly known.

11.) *The Physician Who Saved Bismarck and Established the First Nature Cure Hospital*
Ernest Schweninger (1850-1924) became famous as Otto von Bismarck's personal physician. Schweninger was the son of a respected country doctor, he began his medical studies when he was 16 years old and became a physician at the age of 20. He started out in the field of pathology and became convinced that any cure was ultimately dependent on the healing power of nature. "He did not select nature cure so much as arrived at it through his own evaluation of the processes of disease and cure." (Brauchle 1951)

Schweninger did not want to be the chief physician of a private sanatorium catering to rich, chronically ill patients. He wanted to treat poor patients suffering from acute diseases in a public hospital. In his hospital he avoided surgery and medicine as much as possible, focusing on physical-dietetic treatment like sun, light, air, water, movement, rest, simple diet and psychological influences.

12.) *The First University Professor for Nature Cure Methods.*
Franz Schoenenberger (1865-1933) was the director of the Priessnitz Hospital Berlin Mahlow, it was established in 1927 as the second nature cure hospital.

> *"In the Priessnitz-Hospital we want to put the innate healing power of nature into the physician's command for the benefit of the sick. We hope to prove that natural methods are reliable and successful even in life— threatening diseases. The hospital shall be a research center for nature cure. Its staff will test and confirm scientifically what the ingenious instinct of Priessnitz discovered many decades ago."* (Brauchle 1937)

When Schoenenberger entered the University of Berlin as a student in 1894, he received his doctor's degree in 1898. The title of his dissertation, "*The Influence of Light on the Animal Organism*" including "*Investigations about the Changes of Blood during the Removal of Light*", shows that Schoenenberger focused his research on a subject relevant to nature cure. In 1920 the Prussian minister for culture and education, Konrad Haenisch, appointed Schoenenberger as professor and Head of the Hydrotherapeutic University Institute. Schoenenberger changed the name of the institute to "University Clinic for Natural Living and Healing". The main focus on prevention and nature cure methods had never been seen in a university setting. The clinic offered an ambulatory department with treatment rooms and a small in-patient ward with 20 beds.

> "During nine years, 25,000 patients received repeated counseling and treatment. Approximately 100 women and 50 men were treated daily in the baths. 250,000 baths were administered and 56,000 patients visited the electrotherapy department. In 1921 the department for therapeutic gymnastics and massage was established and carried out 4,500 treatments within 8 years. (Brauchle 1937)

Schoenenberger became the chief physician for the Priessnitz hospital in 1927 but resigned in April of 1929 from this position because of its burden. He did retain his university clinic position until his death on June 7, 1933.

13.) *Cooperation Between Natural and Ortodox Medicine*
Alfred Brauchle (1898-1964) became the director of the Priessnitz Hospital from 1929 till 1935. He had assisted Franz Schoenenberger before, like other nature doctors Brauchle wrote a number of books on natural healing. During his work at the Priessnitz Hospital he wrote one of the first nature cure textbooks specifically for physicians. "*Handbook of Nature Cure on a Scientific Basis.*" (1933)
"*Nature Cure in Biographies*" (1937)
"*Fundamentals of Normal Histological and Microscopic Anatomy* (1925)

In 1957, he wrote *"The Great Book of Nature Cure"* for general public. Brauchle was a member of the Research council of the Emerson University, Los Angeles; Honorary Member of the American Balneological Society. He received the Swiss Rikli Honor Award and the Hufeland Medal.

14.) *The Father of Naturopathy*

Benedict Lust (1872-1945) largely influenced the development of Naturopathy in America by combining nature cure with homeopathy, massage, spinal manipulation, and therapeutic electricity. Nature Cure, consisting of hydrotherapy, air and light baths, a vegetarian diet, and herbal remedies originated in Europe. Lust was born in Michelbach, Germany and came to America in 1892. When he came down with a serious case of tuberculosis, which did not seem to improve despite the best efforts of homeopathy and allopathy. Finally he was given up to die by American doctors. He decided to return to Germany to die in his homeland. Back in Germany, he was able to visit Sebastian Kneipp in Woerishfen. Kneipp looked at him and said: "I don't know if I can put you back together again, but I will see what I can do." Lust's health improved immediately with the Kneipp Cure and he completely recovered in eight months. In 1896 Lust had an audience with Kneipp where he was authorized to bring the Kneipp methods to America as Kneipp's official representative. This was the start of naturopathy in America. At that time, a number of Kneipp institutions had been in existence mainly within German-speaking immigrant communities in New York where Lust settled. But he was the first to be commissioned by Kneipp as well as the first who started to Americanize Kneippism by combining it with other nature cure practices. From the very beginning Lust was persecuted by the New York County Medical Association. By the end of the prosecution Lust had been arrested 16 times by New York authorities and 3 times by federal authorities. This gave rise to the adoption of the term "naturopathy" a term originally coined in 1892 by Dr. John Scheel a water—curist and his wife Sophie Scheel, a homeopath. The Scheels had opened the "Badekur", one of the first water cure institutions in New York. In 1896, they gave Lust the right to use the name "Naturopathy". This was the magic term to end the persecution because words like cure, healing, therapy, therapist, physician, and doctor were prohibited for the nature cure practitioners. Despite being a misnomer "Naturopathy" covered the subject. Lust also defended the criticized combination of a Latin root (nature) with a Greek root (pathos) as intended because "Naturopathy" is supposed to be a hybrid word. Lust's "therapeutic universalism" had the disadvantage that he was burdened with the demanding task of wanting to be knowledgeable in all healing methods resulting in the fact that he did not become a true master in any of them.

To take care of his two "Jungborn' in New Jersey and Florida he became famous as one of the original "frequent flyers". The German government honored him with a gold medal "for distinguished services rendered to mankind", bringing nature cure and drugless therapy to the United States.

15.) *The Matriarch of Naturopathy*
(Aloysia Stroebele) Louisa Lust (1868-1925) had studied nature cure methods of Rikli and Kuhne in London before she came to America. During the early 1890's she was doctor in charge of the Bellevue Sanatorium, a nature cure retreat in Butler, New Jersey, later she was in charge of the women's department at the "Jungborn" retreats in New Jersey and Florida, modeled after the German nature cure institution in the Hartz mountains founded by Adolf Just. Benedict Lust married Louisa in 1901. Louisa was not only "the greatest women doctor in the entire history of the naturopathic movement," she was also a strict promoter of a healthy diet. Her "Practical Naturopathic-Vegetarian Cook Book", the first strictly naturopathic guide for food preparations was popular and influential.

"A large part of food among Americans is composed of white flour, sugar, and butter. People who are living on such stuff are gradually starving themselves to death"

—(L. Lust 1907)

"A minimum of food means a minimum of digestive work. A nervous breakdown is more often traced to overwork of the digestive tract, than the mental apparatus"

—(L. Lust 1924)

"Good housekeeping is the science of combining perfect cleanliness with economy and comfort, careful and intelligent attention to sanitation and the laws of hygiene."

—(L. Lust 1907)

Despite her beliefs she never recommended radical changes to her patients, one step at a time, slowly but surely. Louisa Lust was also a strong advocate of hydrotherapy, she wrote: "If all people understood how to use water, one half of all the afflictions from disease would be removed and the other half would be taken care of by understanding *how and when to eat*." (1911) Together with her husband, she helped to establish the "Jungborn" institutes as well as the first naturopathic college, the American College of Naturopathy in New York where she was the "Instructor of Practical Naturopathy".

Louisa Lust died unexpectedly in 1925 at the age of 57 of "chronic endocarditis".

16.) *Founder of Scientific Naturopathy*
Henry Lindlahr (1862-1924), his transition from a business tycoon to a scientific nature doctor is a quite absorbing story. He was born in Germany and lived there for his first twenty years. He was trained as a brewing and baking chemist, but after his immigration to America he became a respected businessman. He made his fortune in land speculations when he suddenly was diagnosed with diabetes. None of the medical doctors were able to improve his situation. Lindlahr stated: "At the age of thirty-five I found myself as a physical and mental wreck without faith in God, in nature, or myself.

When a friend gave him a copy of Louis Kuhne's book "The Science of Healing" he started to understand the concept of disease being caused by violations of nature's laws. He immediately followed Kuhne's regimen and improved quite drastically but yet his diabetes was still dominant. Lindlahr now decided to seek help in Vienna, but none of the most noted European physicians could help him so now he decided to visit Father Kneipp. Kneipp smelled his breath, surveyed his 250-odd pounds and said bluntly:
　　"You have the sugar disease." "You are a pig" "You will take sitz baths, live
　　on fruits, greens, and vegetables alone. No breads, no cereals, no meats."

By the next spring Lindlahr was free of sugar, had lost 43 pounds and fully recuperated. Back in America, he started a successful nature cure practice in Chicago as a licensed drugless practitioner. Now at the age of forty he decided to study medicine in Chicago and graduated in 1904 from medical school and began to practice full time under his medical license. For the next twenty years he became the foremost practitioner of scientific naturopathy in America. He believed that germs were not the cause of infectious disease but rather secondary manifestation of a disturbed metabolic environment. His early training as a brewery and bakery chemist introduced him to the concept that not all germs were bad. Indeed, the brewers and bakers art depended on beneficial strains of microbes. "His approach was not to kill the germs but rather remove the morbid matter upon which they thrived." In his "Catechism of Nature Cure" Lindlahr later recognized five categories of natural therapy:
1.) Return to Nature　　　　2.) Elementary Remedies
3.) Chemical Remedies　　　4.) Mechanical Remedies
5.) Mental/Spiritual Remedies

17.) *The Inventor of Constitutional Hydrotherapy*
Otis G. Carroll (1879-1962) is remembered for originating constitutional hydrotherapy, a series of hot and cold compresses, the modernized and intensified Priessnitz' wet sheet pack. Carroll was convinced: "If the water treatment fails you, you are doing something wrong". Like the European nature doctors, Carroll believed that disease formed by an overload of toxins in the body, which were frequently the result of faulty digestion. In constitutional hydrotherapy he had a treatment to eliminate toxins as well as an impact in reducing their build up and his constitutional food intolerance test enabled him to prevent the creation of toxin by detecting sensitivities and eliminating such foods out of a patients diet. Dr. Carroll opened his practice 1908 in Spokane, Washington, which he maintained until his death in 1962. He loved his practice and worked day and night with no apparent breaks. One of Carroll's students noted: "He treated germs like they didn't exist", once he had a case of diphtheria. He took a culture, sent it to the state health department and treated the patient. By the time authorities came to quarantine the patient, this patient was well. And they couldn't understand that. (Bastyr 1989) Carroll was also an accomplished herbalist. His botanical remedies in addition to hydrotherapy and nutrition was strongly influenced by Father Kneipp, even though he never personally met him.

18.) *The Scottish Nature Cure Pioneer*
James C Thomson (1887-1960) wrote many books about health and healthy living, he was highly inspired by Dr. Henry Lindlahr when he traveled to America in search of a comprehensive system of natural remedies, based on science and a common philosophy. He quickly adopted Lindlahr beliefs in the "Vis medicatrix naturae" when Lindlahr made him manager of his sanatorium in Chicago. After he returned to Scotland in 1912 he established a small practice in Edinburgh, regarding hydrotherapy as important part of his nature cure practice his recommended applications ranged within the tradition of Priessnitz, Kneipp, and Kuhne. It was no secret that Thomson was obviously against pharmaceuticals, once he was asked during a lecture "What would you put in the place of drugs?" Thomson answered: "Surely if we get rid of a bad thing, it is unnecessary to put anything in its place." Besides his practice he also was the principal of the Edinburgh School of Natural Therapeutics, which he founded in 1913. This was the only place in Britain for a truly professional and adequate training in Nature Cure. Later he established the Society of Registered Naturopaths with the goal to check and support the students who graduated from the Edinburgh School and help them to build good practices.

19.) *England's Foremost Naturopath*
Stanley Lief (1892-1963) and James C. Thomson created the standard for naturopathy in Britain like Lust and Lindlahr in America. Lief traveled to America to enroll at Macfadden's International College of Drugless Physicians in Chicago. Before he returned to England he also visited Henry Lindlahr. Back home he became manager of Macfadden's "Healthatorium" at Brighton. After the war Lief purchased Champneys to turn this elegant estate into the first natural health retreat in England, which finally became the largest nature cure establishment in the world. Like Otis G. Carroll he regarded germs not as primary cause, but as secondary manifestation of disease. He also considered disease as a systematic disturbance requiring the treatment of the whole patient. *"No ailment is produced in the body by chance nor is it caused by an outside influence. Ill-health always arises from a condition within the body"* (Lief 1931)
Lief's 5-point plan for treating colds:
"Stop eating; flush the bowels; take warm baths; get plenty of fresh air and rest in bed." This strategy was applied to most problems. Lief was also known to be very strict: *"When I say daily regime, I mean 365 days in a year"* Traveling the world to investigate new natural treatments, his basic message was:
"There are no substitutes for obedience to the never changing laws of life" (Lief 1963) Lief actively contributed to the growth of naturopathy in Great Britain. In 1938 he was able to open the Nature Cure Association and clinic, which became the still present British College of Naturopathy and Osteopathy. It was destroyed in World War II and rebuilt at its present site in Hempstead.

20.) *Canada's International Ambassador for Naturopathy*
Arno R. Koegler (1898-1991) like many of the early nature doctors, he was born in Germany and deeply inspired by Emmanuel Felke, who brought him back to health after a terrible train accident. In 1923 Koegler, his wife, and two children immigrated to Canada where he opened a naturopathic practice in 1926 in Waterloo, Ontario, he was a teacher at the Canadian Memorial Chiropractic College where he trained the founding members of the Board of the Ontario College of Naturopathic Medicine established in 1978. In 1956 Koegler became president of the International Society of Naturopathic Physicians (ISNP) until 1972. He also was president of the International Council on Homeopathy. One of Koegler's favorite sayings was:" As long as there are medical doctors around, there will be lots of work" (Bander 1991) Koegler received the "Prix Hippocrate" in Paris for his research work in natural medicine and was appointed Honorary Professor of Botanical Medicine at the University in Barcelona, he went to South America, New Zealand, and Australia and even met the queen of England.

21.) *An Inspiring Teacher of Naturopathy from Canada*
Joseph A. Boucher (1916-1987) even though a Canadian he played an important role in the development of naturopathy in the United States. In 1956, he joined John Bastyr and others in founding the National College of Naturopathic Medicine in Seattle. After the college moved to Portland, Boucher traveled there every Friday to teach his classes for many years. "Joseph Boucher is not remembered for new diagnostic therapeutic techniques or revolutionizing naturopathic practice. He is remembered because his "strong shoulders and gentle heart helped carry naturopathy through some of its hardest years." (Matsen 1987)

22.) *Father of Modern Naturopathic Medicine*
John Bastyr (1912-1995) observed his basic skills at an early age by helping his father in his pharmacy and observing his mother's gardening skills and her knowledge as herbalist. She was a true believer in Father Kneipp. In 1936 Bastyr enrolled at Seattle's Drugless Institute. Later he studied homeopathy with C.P. Bryant and occasionally this knowledge became handy while working in his fathers pharmacy. After Bastyr opened his first practice in Seattle, he went to Spokane to study with Dr. Otis G. Carroll after one of his patients whom he had sent there for treatment, came back cured. And somehow in his busy schedule Bastyr still found time to gather and prepare many of his own herbal remedies. When the College of Naturopathic Medicine was founded in Portland in 1956 and moved to Seattle in 1959 Bastyr served as the "Executive Director" and taught obstetrics and gynecology. Later the college moved back to Portland, Oregon because of the more liberal laws toward naturopathy, but requiring weekly journeys for their teaching naturopathic doctors. In 1978 the John Bastyr College of Naturopathic Medicine, now Bastyr University was founded in Seattle by Bastyr's former students, Joseph E. Pizzorno and William Mitchell, to carry on the educational heritage of their mentor. Nowadays Bastyr considers his allopathic colleagues more tolerant and appreciative of naturopathic methods.

"I remember when we would give a diet to a patient, and the medical men would just laugh" (Bastyr 1989)

Bastyr saw the medical knowledge increase in both allopathy and naturopathy and played a major role to assure the integration of the latest findings from scientific literature into naturopathic medical education.

Even though it may seem strange to have a "laudatio" appear as addendum of the first chapter, I would like to express my special thanks to Friedhelm Kirchfeld, librarian at the College of Naturopathic Medicine in Portland, Oregon and author of the book "Nature Doctors". He generously allowed me to use extracts from his book for my hydrotherapy classes. As I mentioned my segment of Nature Doctors is just an extract of essentials. The abundance of information and stories in Friedhelm Kirchfeld's book, "Nature Doctors", is a documentation of tremendous research, entertaining and educational.

LEVEL 1/CHAPTER II

History of Balneology

Balneology, the science about medicinal uses of mineral and thermal water developed in the 2nd half of the 19th century, even though first chemical analysis of mineral waters were reported at the end of the 18th century. In the beginning of the 20th century, laboratories and institutes became interested in spas, allowing a more scientific examination of the patients and supervision of treatment results. A growing number of doctors settled within spas and engaged in empirical investigations of cure remedies and their effects. Documentations about Hydro-and Balneotherapy for therapeutic purposes came from France, England, and Germany around the 17th century.

The therapeutic application of spring-water or mineral water is referred to as "Crenotherapy". Crenology involves the science of mineral springs their chemical composition as well as temperature and location. Balneotherapy is the therapeutic application of bath (partial-, half-, full-) with or without herbal or mineral extracts, gas, peloids, mud or clay including drinking of mineral water or inhalation. Hydrotherapy is the use of water with dietetic, prophylactic, or therapeutic purpose in all thermal stages from steam to ice.

Medicinal Bath Therapy distinguishes 3 categories:

 a.) synthetic medicinal baths

 b.) bath with phytoextracts

 c.) special medicinal baths colon hydrotherapy, four-cell-bath/Hydro-electric baths.

Water as supra-natural property

As most abundant and useful substance water covers more than 70% of the earth's surface and also exists as vapor in the earth's atmosphere. It is essential to life not only by assisting homeostasis inside the human body; it also influences weather and climate. (Medical Hydrology and Climatology) Almost all chemical reactions seem to require water. A molecule of pure water consists of two atoms of hydrogen (H) and one atom of oxygen (O) = H_2O.

To break down a water molecule H_2O you *don't get* H+ H+ O it chemically breaks down into H (Hydrogen ion) and OH (Hydroxide ion). Basically one hydrogen atom is left alone, and the other hydrogen atom gets the oxygen, which creates one positive ion and one negative ion. The hydrogen ion helps to create acids and the hydroxide ion helps to create bases. Since water is a combination of two different elements (hydrogen and oxygen) it is considered a compound. Compounds are formed when molecules of two or more atoms are joined together. Several atoms of carbon, hydrogen, and oxygen = glucose=$C_6H_{12}O_6$.

"Pure Water is a tasteless, odorless liquid. One gallon of water weighs about 8.3 pounds, one liter weighs 1 kilogram. Water is regarded as incompressible, which is a valuable property for Hydraulics.

Water is a great solvent, dissolving more particles than any other known substance. For this reason pure water is never found in nature! Water in lakes, rivers, and wells always contains minerals dissolved from the earth. Rainwater contains chemicals dissolved from the air. Pure water can only be obtained by distillation. Ground water as natural reservoir in sand, gravel, porous rocks, and cavities under the ground, feeds springs, wells, rivers, even the ocean.

A spring can be classified as "therapeutic" if it contains a minimum of one or more minerals per liter water.
A Japanese spring has to flow from the earth at a minimum temperature of 77 F and is supposed to contain a minimum amount of at least one of the following components:
Free carbon dioxide (1000 mg.)
Copper (1 mg.)
Iron (20 mg.)
Aluminum (100 mg)
Hydrogen (1 mg.)
Arsenic (0.7 mg)
Sulfur (2mg)
Radon (8.25 mache units)

The presence of specific minerals and gases determine the medicinal qualities of a spring. The unusual combination of free carbon dioxide with sodium chloride and bicarbonates of sodium, calcium and magnesium made Saratoga Springs, New York popular for treating heart disease, arthritis, and skin problems in the nineteenth and beginning 20th century. Mineral springs containing sulfur and sulfates are considered antibacterial and antifungal.

Water for Consumption

Surface water may be polluted by sewage, industrial wastes, dead plants or animals. Groundwater may be polluted by sewage or industrial wastes leaking into the ground. Surface and ground water can also contain silt and other solids creating objectionable tastes and odors. Communities with a high quality source of water may be able to distribute it right from the source, while others may need to purify the water before distribution. If chlorine is used as disinfectant, activated carbon or ammonia is usually also added to remove the chlorine taste from the water.

Many religions imply symbolic meanings onto water. In Christian Baptism, water is used to symbolize the washing away of sin. According to Jewish beliefs, water is a symbol of purity. To Hindus, it is a symbol of fertility and Taoists regard water as the symbol of humility because it always seeks the lowest place.

17th Century: Dawn of Scientific Interest

Even though it is known that spring and mineral waters have been used for thousands of years it was not until the 18th century that spa waters became of scientific interest. In 1737, the first documentation about the usefulness of mineral waters had been published.

When mineral springs experienced growing appreciation in Japan, their given names identified their specific curative properties. Physicians from China and Japan started to evaluate and classify several medicinal springs. The first medical study of hot springs in Tokyo was conducted in 1709.

By the 17th century there was an abundance of spas throughout Europe, which also indicated a growing interest in the medicinal value of mineral springs. During the 18th and 19th century many European spas were meticulously studied and evaluated by chemists. Physicians developed treatment protocols for a variety of health disorders. Until today specialized spa treatment prescribed by physicians are covered by all health insurances. Some European spas are affiliated with universities and medical schools staffed by trained medical specialists.

Interest in mineral springs in America developed soon after European colonists arrived and learned about the many springs Native Americans considered sacred. Many of the larger mineral spring resorts were modeled after the famous European spas. Medicinal properties of spas became of interest at the end of the 18th century in America. During the 19th century, chemists and physicians analyzed and classified hundreds of North American mineral and thermal springs. Numerous types of water applications were introduced from Europe. Hydrotherapy was offered in private, state, and federal hospitals. Dr. Simon Baruch, Professor of Balneology at the College of Physicians at Columbia University published his book *"Use of Water in Modern Medicine"* in 1893. The Simon Baruch Research Institute established in 1933 at Saratoga Spa was the first institute for balneological research in the United States. By the 1900s hydrotherapy was well integrated in to medical treatments and part of orthopedic hospitals. Unfortunately, by the end of the 19th century this interest faded in America when more sophisticated scientific medicine made balneotherapy seem old fashioned and gradually the medical community lost interest in the therapeutic value of spa treatments.

The Simon Baruch Research Institute finally had to close because of insufficient funding. While water therapy remained popular in Europe and Japan, America and Britain had lost interest in the medicinal value of mineral and thermal water, mainly because it lacked objective scientific proof.

The medical research conducted at the Simon Baruch Research Institute focused mainly on cardiology and rheumatology until its closing.
European physicians who conducted research in balneology viewed water not as experimental drug. They considered the denial of a beneficial therapy to a patient as unethical. Bathing in thermal and mineral springs has been medically recommended for hundreds of years. And properly applied water therapies have been proven safe and effective for millions of people. This approach is in consent with German health insurances who fully cover physiotherapy if prescribed by a physician for rehabilitative and preventative purposes.

Leading universities and spa-based scientific organizations:

o   International Society of Medical Hydrology and Climatology
o   German Society of Health Resort Medicine and Spa Treatment

o German Society for Balneology and Climatology/Technical University Munich

o Austrian Society for Balneology and Bioclimatology/University of Vienna

o Institute of Medical Balneology and Climatology of the Ludwig—Maximilians University Munich

o University of Innsbruck

o Paracelsus Society Bad Hall.

Because of the importance of Bad Hall main research subjects: "Basic Research on iodine, antioxidative defense mechanisms and their role in prevention and rehabilitation, especially in cardiovascular and eye diseases, as well as general balneologic investigation with the goal to prove the efficiency of the iodine brine," I am briefly going to explain the importance of iodine in the following segment.

1811 accidental discovery of iodine

Iodine-containing remedies like ash of seaweed or roasted sponge were recommended against goiter long before the knowledge of the element iodine. The iodine waters of Bad Hall were sold and used for baking "Kropfbrot" (goiter bread). The essential trace element iodine was discovered by accident in 1811 by producing lime of salpetre from seaweed. It became utilized as a goiter remedy in 1816. Commercially iodine is obtained from Caliche, a Chilean nitrate—bearing earth and from seaweed ash. Iodine is prepared by displacement of an iodine compound with chlorine. It is a shiny bluish-black solid, which volatizes at ordinary temperatures into an irritating blue-violet gas. Iodine is the essential component of the two thyroid hormones T4 and T3. The daily-required iodine amount lies between 150 and 300 µg. 5 grams of iodized common salt will get you 80 µg of iodine. Natural sources of iodine are sea fish, kiwi, mahaleb cherry juice concentrates, and iodine rich mineral waters like those in Bad Hall containing ~ 40 mg/L. Iodine deficiencies during pregnancy can lead to mental retardation, stunted growth, and hearing defects. Iodine is important in all degenerative diseases especially arteriosclerosis, diabetes, mellitus, and joint diseases.

Iodine effects beyond the thyroid:

Iodine as an antiseptic:

• Antibacterial

- Antiviral
- Antifungal

Iodine as a secretolytic in the Respiratory Tract

Iodine and connective tissue:
- loosening (swelling)
- favorable effects on: collagen synthesis (wound healing),
- blood vessels (against arteriosclerosis)
- cartilage (against arthroses)
- eye media

Iodine effects on the eye
- opacities of the vitreous body
- "dry eye"
- macular degeneration at the beginning
- incipient cataract

Indications for the treatments offered in Bad Hall

Eye Diseases
Degenerative alterations of the eye background, esp. initial stages of macular degeneration, consecutive conditions of high myopia (opacity of the vitreous body, degeneration of the retina) vascular diseases (e.g. in connection with hypertension; diabetes)
Affections of the optic nerve
Incipient cataract
So-called "dry eye"
chronic conjunctivitis and inflammation of the margin of the eyelid.

Arteriosclerosis
Angina pectoris
Stroke
Smoker's leg
Hypertension
Parkinson's Disease
Affections of the Backbone
Disorders of the intervertebral disks

Treatment after joint replacement and operation of vertebral disks.
Osteoporosis
Phantom-limb pain

LEVEL I/CHAPTER III

The origin of Phytotherapy

Aromatic plants and fragrant flowers are some of nature's most beautiful creations. Fragrances from flowers, leaves, roots, seeds, and woods are an important part of every culture as medicine, foods, spices, perfumes, and incense. The distillation of essential oil evolved over at least 4,000 years. The simple methods used for extracting botanical materials from plants guided the way towards herbal preparations. In medieval Europe, country people had always gathered wild useful plants; but it was in the monastic herb gardens that plants of known virtue were transplanted and organized in beds and their usefulness studied and catalogued. Herbs were being cultivated in Europe, not just for their availability when needed but also to be enjoyed as amenity. The old herbal wisdom started to decline in the nineteenth century and now modern gardeners need to release their instinctive affinity with herbs. Alternative medicine is rediscovering some of the skills of phytotherapy and the abundance of applications. The earliest scientific documentation came from Theophrastus: "*Enquiry into plants and Growth of Plants*" (300 BC)
Avicenna: "*Canon Medicinae*" (1920)
Leech: "*Book of Bald*" (950)

The botanist refers to an herb as a plant that dies down to the ground at the end of the growing season. A medicinal herb is considered a plant that assists in the prevention or treatment of illness; whereas, the cook refers to an herb as part of a plant used in preparation of food.

The collection of aromatic herbs can be traced back as far as ancient Egypt.

Notable Herb Flowers
- Borage—rich blue; for salads and summer drinking
- Lavender—soft purple; for scent and pot-pourri

- Nasturtiums—vivid reds and yellows; for colored garnishes
- Violets—purple; for medicines and crystallized as decoration
- Elderflowers—white and fragrant; for wines, cordials, and flavoring fruit dishes
- Pot marigolds or calendulas—vivid orange; for salads, pot-pourri, and food coloring
- Rose petals—red roses of scented varieties; for color and fragrance, wines, and perfumes
- Woodruff—tiny and white; imparts scent of hay and vanilla when warm

Although the fragrance of herbs is the main reason for their cultivation, in many cases the scent represents the metabolic waste products of the plant. Substances like geraniol in roses or thyme and eucalyptol in thyme are essential oils formed within the plant, and then stored in cells near the leaf surfaces. Pressure or movement, such as that of a browsing animal, a strong breeze, or the heat of the sunlight will release these chemicals to defend or shield the plant from injury.

Many plants produce natural insecticides as part of their defense system. Various Tagetes species are known to repel whitefly infestation and other pests when grown in greenhouses. Scientific research confirms that their flowers emit volatile chemicals into the surrounding air for protection. The same chemicals have been proven to be toxic to mosquitoes and, hopefully, a new generation of insecticides can be developed.

All plants are complex factories producing diverse chemicals and any of these substances may be harmful in particular circumstances. The medical benefits of herbs are no longer in doubt and most are quite safe, provided that they are not misused or taken when allergic reactions are known. Herbs interact in complex ways with our body's chemistry. Compared to synthetic drugs their actions may seem very mild; yet, do not underestimate the danger of self-medication on the assumption that herbs are harmless. Herbalists positively revel in the chemical complexity of even the simplest plant, realizing that it is in this very multiplicity of chemical components that the strength of the herb arises and from where it draws its healing virtue. Some plant constituents buffer the action of other potent plant chemicals to prevent possible harmful side effects. Looking at "Rauwolfia Serpentina", famous for its alkaloid reserpine, the whole plant contains at least 160 additional alkaloids, some of which have a balancing or buffering effect on reserpine.

To harvest herbs correctly and preserve the plants beneficial properties, you will have to gather them at the right moment during the day and the right point in the growing season. To harvest leaves for their medicinal value it is best to gather them when the flowers are in bud and before any have opened. It should be done early in the day, as soon as the dew has evaporated from the plant. Flowers should be picked, also, early in the day as soon as possible after they are fully open. Roots should be harvested at the end of the growing season when maximum amounts of nutrients are stored there in preparation for the winter.

Medicinal herbs have been used also in baths for many centuries, with the distinction between cosmetic and medicinal use. It has been proven that herbal bath extracts greatly enhance skin stimulation besides the percutaneous absorption of plant constituents. Father Sebastian Kneipp is credited for rediscovering medical herbs.

1.) Kneippism:

Kneipp supporters represent the largest group of individuals active in European health movement. There are more than 660 clubs of the Kneipp society with approximately 160,000 members. "Kneippism" has become a way of life for many people returning to a healthier lifestyle as philosophy. The combination of warm and cold water, fresh air, sunlight, and herbs along with diet and exercise is used to nurture and strengthen the mind, soul, and body. Father Kneipp believed that if our mode of life can have a detrimental effect on our health, than a change in this mode of life can restore it. Kneipp's holistic science of health is based on five elements:

1.) Hydrotherapy; comforting and strengthening:

Water serves as mediator for temperature stimuli causing vascular, muscular, and metabolic responses. The simplest forms of Kneipp—hydrotherapy are walking barefoot in the morning dew, treading water in a brook, stream or bathtub and jogging in the snow.

2.) Phytotherapy

Herbal extracts are used to stimulate the body's defense mechanism and to increase the benefits of a particular water application. Scientific research has proven that essential oils added to the bath water penetrate through the skin and are able to unfold their calming or stimulating effects on the body. Plant extracts can be used either curative or preventative.

3.) Kinesi Therapy/Exercise

Aerobic exercise amplifies the energizing effect of water stimuli and the supportive influence of herbs. Physical activity also increases mental efficiency, while promoting mental and psychological relaxation.

4.) Dietetic Therapy
Kneipp's natural nutrition philosophy, a well balanced diet with healthful nutrients rich in vitamins, low in fat and sugar.
5.) Regulative Therapy
Lifestyle—harmony of body, mind, and soul:
According to Kneipp the equanimity of the soul is a prerequisite for physical well being, an active way of life leads to harmony of body, mind, and soul; but whatever constitutes this activity is up to the individual. Reading, painting, hobbies, exercise, mediation, prayer, relaxation exercises are equally valid.

2.) The Redefined Kneipp System

The Kneipp water applications are based on the findings of Vincent Priessnitz who only used cold-water treatments. Having used those therapies to cure his own ailments, Kneipp realized that a such harsh regime might not be suitable for everybody so he adapted his applications, modified and redefined them until he developed a system that was simple to maintain as a permanent routine in daily life.

The Kneipp treatment or Kneipp Kur is a specific hydrotherapeutic program that also includes a natural food diet, exercise, and herbs. The techniques applied are ablutions alternating between hot and cold water as well as washing the entire body with warm water every 20 or 30 minutes to induce perspiration. Kneipp recommended arm, leg, and foot baths, hot and cold packs as well as compresses to specific parts of the body, affusions from an unnozzled hose or watering can of differing temperatures and pressures followed by 10 minutes of exercise to increase circulation. Each affusion is applied according to a prescribed sequence but all begin at the most distant point of the heart. For a contrast affusion begin with a warm spray right and left followed immediately with a cold spray both sides and repeat warm right and left. Written in the text book "Medical Balneology" by Dr. Kurt Franke a morning program for a four week Kneipp Kur looks like this:
First treatment between 6 and 7 a.m. could be an ablution of the trunk or a dry brushing of the skin followed by a cool after-ablution. This maybe applied in bed. Early morning wading in the dewy grass for one to five minutes or in the winter a 1/2 to 1 minute walk in the snow (barefoot of course). Later in the morning, stronger applications are given in the hydrotherapy department. Like contrast foot-

bath, knee affusions, cold affusion to the upper thigh and back as well as herbal bath if indicated.

Note that cold applications like snow-wading cold gushes, spritz gush, blitz gush are performed very brief to stimulate the autonomic nerve receptors, half a minute is plenty; you don't want to over stimulate.

The diet is mostly plant oriented, rich in vitamins, low in fat, whole wheat bread, and fresh raw vegetables. One major ingredient of Kneipp therapeutic recommendations during the Kneipp Kur is the "Regulative—or Order Therapy". Most people will associate Kneipp with cold water, which is just one small link within the chain. The regulative therapy is meant to take home and maybe become your philosophy for balanced lifestyle.

How often do you get upset looking for something important you "misplaced", how much time does it cost you to be "sloppy"? Wouldn't it be much easier to find things if you would have put them right where they belonged, so you don't have to stress yourself to remember where you left the scissors if they were returned to the kitchen drawer. This example can follow you throughout your entire life, without being excessive compulsive or a geek. Your child can put the toys back where they belong, this way they don't break, you would not lose one part of your favorite puzzle, the homework is in your backpack, and so on down to the sock drawer.

If you create a healthy order in your life, you will eliminate a good amount of stress.

As stress accumulates during the day, often beyond our control, we will have to deal with negative impact. We have to find a way to bring balance into our lives and eliminate the stress factors.

By the way, wouldn't it be nice to find your socks immediately in the morning anyways?

While looking at the long list of psychosomatic diseases like:

    Depression
    Exhaustion
    Stomach ulcers
    Diarrhea
    Muscle tension
    Irregular heartbeat

and many more chronic problems you may be able to trace back to permanent stressors.

Level I/Chapter IV

Commercial Influx in 21st Century Hydrotherapy

1.) Health, Wellness, and Beauty
Spa therapies, even in Europe where the main focus was health, rehabilitation or prevention, now offer the complex approach of health, wellness, and cosmetic corrections. In comprehensive spas, you will find oriental massage or traditional Chinese massage as well as acupressure, acupuncture, aromatherapy, body scrubs, Balneotherapy, therapeutic massage, sports massage, oxygen therapy, ozone therapy, sauna, and, of course, spa cuisine which refers to a healthy natural diet from mainly fresh fruits and vegetables, low sodium, no artificial flavorings or preservatives. Thalassotherapy is more specific for spas with ocean access since it includes the inhalation of the air, seawater therapy, and seaweed wraps. Chemically, the ocean is a strong solution of common salt.

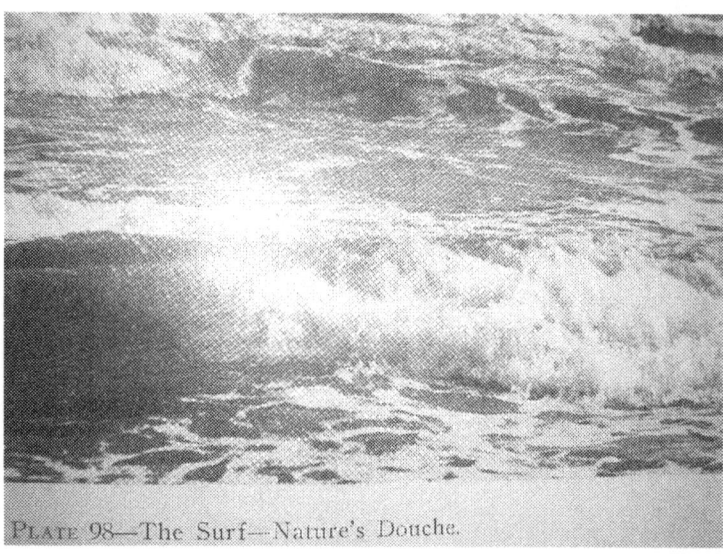

PLATE 98—The Surf—Nature's Douche.

Chloride of sodium..................	25.10
Chloride of potassium..................	.50
Chloride of magnesium...............	3.50
Sulphate of magnesium................	5.78
Sulphate of lime.........................	.15
Carbonate of magnesium.............	.18
Carbonate of lime......................	.02
Carbonate of potassium...............	.23
Iodides and bromides.................	traces
Organic matter.......................	traces
Water................................	964.54
Total:.................................	1,000 mg/l

Hot springs or mineral springs combined with complementary natural therapies enhance their physical, thermal, and chemical effectiveness supported by environmental climatic effects. The general hotel spa guest mostly tends to massage and maybe facials to relief tension after traveling or conference meetings. It is still rare for the United States to plan a spa vacation over a week or two to experience the full benefits of all implementing factors according to Kneipp. As of now, spa therapy is mostly "trauma control" at the end of a stressful event; but the tendency is going towards medi-spa and medically oriented comprehensive treatment facilities for a long-term future establishment beyond fashionable "ins" and "outs".

2.) Europe vs. United States:
Functional Therapeutic vs. Luxurious Entertainment
American and also British spas have a distinct disadvantage compared to European and Japanese spas by lacking medical supervision. The medical spas only recently started to gain interest but more from a commercial aspect. Most American spas focus on cosmetics or relaxation rather than being therapeutic. The functional therapeutic factor has not quite reached the consumer yet, while European spas offer an extensive range of safe, effective, medically supervised therapies recommended for a wide range of health problems. One major roadblock, of course, are American health insurances, which do not cover spa therapies even if the physician would consider them medically beneficial. In Germany, for example all physiotherapies are fully covered by health insurances even as preventative measure. Noting that thousands of Americans travel to European spas every year to improve their health there is definitely a demand for this service. How to establish the accessibility to a larger percentage of

Americans will remain in question as long as there is no health insurance coverage in the United States for these therapies. Until then, American spas will have to be creative to attract potential customers, and hopefully will also find a way to integrate simple, affordable remedies beyond the bare luxury.

3.) The Genesis of Medical Spas in the United States
The treatment trends are toward alternative medical treatment, preventative medicine, as well as "age intervention" and individual "need-related" issues. With growing interest in the lymphatic system and the damaging effects of lymphostasis, there is a wide spectrum of opportunities for medical spa focus. The treatment of lymphedema, lymphostasis, or simple jet lag related fluid retention are most satisfying. America is ready for the shift to the holistic health model of wellness integrating the philosophy of daily rituals and ongoing preventative treatments. The quick fix approach is no longer convincing for the educated consumer. The higher the level of understanding about homeostasis the greater the willingness to participate in curative therapies, personalized spa treatments, and personalized recommendations on nutritional needs.

European spas have always been medically oriented, where treatments are prescribed and monitored by a physician.

Whether the business is called a medical facility or medical practice in the United States, compliance with regulations will be required. The board of medicine in each state will determine if certain equipment can be used by a physician only or under a physicians supervision; for example, 13 states have restricted use of laser for hair removal to physicians only, 7 states are allowed the use of laser by others under direct physicians supervision. More than 20 states do not recognize esthetician licenses in medical practice. Is the medical spa a medical practice or a spa? The state laws vary and will impact how the medical spa operates. If a physician operates out of a medical spa, the consumer is considered a patient not a client. The consumer perceives this as a medical treatment. Licensing requirements requires investigation since it varies from state to state as well as insurance coverage. Regardless of who is licensed for what, if an independent esthetician shares the same waiting room with a physician the physician ultimately carries the responsibility.

Whoever works in a doctor's office becomes the doctor's employee and the doctor is incurring the liability, this creates a challenge for the doctor. The bottom line is not just are you licensed, but are you also properly trained?

How do wellness spas fit into the medical spa equation? At this point, we can play scrabble between "pseudo medical" and "spa-licensed clinic" to "genuine medical spa" and "wellness center". Even though the guidelines still vary from state to state one subject is clear: a medical spa as a facility has to have a full time medical doctor present.

The natural spa is offering natural treatments hands on, whole body therapeutic service without chemicals or artificial tools for the client who wants to avoid chemical products. The focus is on the energy transmitted between therapist and client, the art of touch combined with the pure product. A holistically based spa offers a whole body approach to wellness under a holistic doctors guidance.

Level II:
BALNEOTHERAPY IN THEORY AND PRACTICE

Balneotherapy is considered the therapeutic application of bath (partial-, half-, full-, spray-, gush-, sponge-) with or without herbal or mineral extracts, gas, peloids, mud, clay including inhalation and drinking of specific mineral waters. Because of the important role of water temperature in hydrotherapy, I will repeat a few temperatures and their effects.

- "The water-temperature determines the extent of skin stimulation!"
- The body will respond by increasing or decreasing circulation.
- Never exceed the maximum tolerance temperature (the highest possible temperature tolerable without sustaining damage)
  - 45-46 C/116-120 F in water
  - 100 C/212 F in air

Depending on duration of exposure and percentage of exposed aerial.

- The tolerance temperature in water also changes proportionally:
  - It decreases with increasing amounts of water

Definitions of Water-Temperature

Possibly injurious	50 C	Above 25 F
Painfully hot	42.8-46 C	110-120 F
Very hot	40-42.8 C	104-110 F
Hot	38-40 C	100-104 F
Warm	34-38 C	92-100 F
Tepid	27-34 C	80-92 F
Cool	21-27 C	70-80 F
Cold	13-21 C	55-70 F
Very Cold	0-13 C	32-55 F

Burns at Specific Temperatures

Temperature	Length of exposure	Degree of Burn
158 (70 C)	1 second	full thickness of skin
149 (65 C)	2 seconds	full thickness of skin
140 (60 C)	3.5 seconds	full thickness of skin
135 (57 C)	10 seconds	full thickness of skin
133 (56 C)	15 seconds	full thickness of skin
127 (53 C)	60 seconds	full thickness of skin

Special Responses to Cold and Hot

Cold	Hot
Heart: first fast, then slow	*Heart*: first slow, then fast

Vessels: the action, contraction; the reaction, dilation
Nerves: numbing
Muscles: reduces volume
Respiration: slows and deepens
Stomach: increases hydrochloric acid and motion
Blood: increases blood count, both RBC's (30-50%) and WBC's (15-50%), increases phagocytosis unless prolonged to chilling
Kidneys: congests and stimulates
Metabolism: increases CO_2; decreases urea; improves oxidation

Vessels: the action, dilation; the reaction; contraction when intense
Nerves: excites
Muscles: increases volume
Respiration: quickens
Stomach: decreases hydrochloric acid and motion
Blood: increases blood count, both RBC's and WBC's, increases phagocytosis
Kidneys: reduces activity
Metabolism: decreases CO_2 in the blood by over breathing; increases urea and general protein wastes

Conversion Table
Temperature

F	C	C	F
0	-17.8	0	32.0
95	35.0	35.0	95.0
96	35.6	35.5	95.9
97	36.1	36.0	96.8
98	36.7	36.5	97.7
99	37.2	37.0	98.6
100	37.8	37.5	99.5
101	38.3	38.0	100.4
102	38.9	38.5	101.3
103	39.4	39.0	102.2
104	40.0	39.5	103.1
105	40.6	40.0	104.0
106	41.1	40.5	104.9
107	41.7	41.0	105.8
108	42.2	41.5	106.7
109	42.8	42.0	107.8
110	43.3	100	212

The Celsius scale has 100 steps compared to the Fahrenheit scale with 180 steps.
The bigger C-scale is 9/5 the size of the F-scale (5/9).
To change Celsius into Fahrenheit multiply by 9/5 + 32 and to change Fahrenheit to Celsius subtract 32 and multiply the rest by 5/9.

LEVEL II/CHAPTER I

Essentials for Hydrotherapy

- *Contents of Water*

Water as tasteless, odorless liquid is never found uncontaminated in nature. "Pure Water" can only be obtained by distillation.

Since water is such a great solvent, it dissolves traces of everything it comes in contact with.

Even rainwater contains chemicals dissolved from the air, and in ground water or springs we find minerals and trace elements like bicarbonate, calcium, chloride, magnesium, nitrate, potassium, sodium, sulfate, lithium, fluoride, and more based upon the location.

The documentation of minerals and trace minerals in spring water applies for bathing as well as bottled water for consumption. Depending on the country of origin the measurements are given in milligrams per liter, parts per million, or milligrams per kilogram.

Seawater contains a mixture of sodium chloride, potassium chloride, magnesium chloride, magnesium sulphate, Sulphate of lime, magnesium carbonate, carbonate of lime, potassium carbonate, iodides and bromides.

The medicinal qualities of water are determined by the amount of specific minerals and gases as well as the temperature of springs.

- *Bicarbonate*

We differentiate between two kinds of bicarbonates resulting from an incomplete neutralization of carbonic acid. (Calcium bicarbonate and sodium bicarbonate)

Sodium bicarbonate or bicarbonate of soda ($NaHCO_3$) = baking soda = is known to relieve stomach acidity

- *Calcium Bicarbonate*

Ca $(HCO_3)_2$ = calcium carbonate + carbonic acid + water is easily soluble and can be directly taken up by plants and animals. The absorbed calcium bicar-

bonate is then integrated into the skeleton. This process is changing calcium bicarbonate back to calcium carbonate (Ca CO_3), releasing CO_2.
Calcium carbonate is not soluble by itself. (It is commonly used in toothpaste and stomach medications.)

European spas, recommended for gastric disorders are located around springs with high bicarbonate content. Due to the anti-inflammatory and antispasmodic effect usually 200 milliliters of carbonated water are suggested as a drink an hour before meals.
As bath-therapy baking soda baths are also commonly known as detox baths. Based on the patient's condition 3 to 5 baths per week may be indicated in 95-100 degrees F for 5 to 15 minutes.

- *Chloride*

Chemical compound of chlorine (Cl) or chemical salt is a compound formed by a chemical reaction between an acid and a base.
The total neutralization of an acid creates a "normal" salt.
If the neutralization is incomplete, an acid salt or basic salt is produced.
Seawater or salt water springs often contain a mixture of sodium chloride (NaCL), potassium chloride, calcium chloride, and magnesium chloride.
The healing properties of salt water springs are usually determined by the dominance of a specific chloride. High concentrations of sodium chloride are also considered brine waters. Brine bathing is praised in many well-known European spas. Only a few chloride rich springs are also found in the United States. Bathing is recommended for recuperation after trauma from accidents or surgery, skin problems, problems of the central and peripheral nervous system and gynecological disorders.
Drinking of these waters is commonly prescribed for a variety of symptoms as well as inhalation therapy for respiratory infections.

- *Sulfur (s)*

Sulfur springs contain free hydrogen sulfide, which is responsible for the strong odor. Sulfur has been known for thousands of years, in the Bible it was referred to as brimstone. Bathing in sulfur-rich springs is recommended for several health problems from urinary tract conditions to rheumatism, chronic skin diseases even heavy metal poisoning.
The released hydrogen sulfide gas possesses strong antibacterial properties and is known to relieve respiratory problems.

When inhalation therapy is prescribed it can be administered by a nebulizer in form of a fine mist or as sulfur bath water where the evaporating vapors are inhaled.

- **Sulfates**

Chemical mixture of sulfur and oxygen usually formed in crystals (Epson salt). Other chemical compositions are:
Calcium sulfate, sodium sulfate, magnesium sulfate. Bathing in magnesium sulfate is known to soothe and tighten the skin as well as allowing it to retain moisture.

- **Gases**

Some mineral waters contain carbon dioxide or radon.
Carbon dioxide (CO_2) is colorless, odorless, incombustible gas, consisting of 1 carbon atom and 2 oxygen atoms. It is formed during respiration as waste product of the body and is used by plants during photosynthesis transforming carbon dioxide into oxygen.
Carbonated waters are characterized by tiny bubbles of carbon dioxide. Those waters are prescribed for bathing as well as drinking mainly for circulatory problems, arthritis, and cardiovascular disorders.
During a 4-week program the patient receives approximately 20—bath treatments beginning at 5 minutes in 34 C (94 F) in slightly diluted carbon dioxide water.

After the third bath the duration is increased to 10 minutes with a20% carbon dioxide saturation. Towards the end of the treatments, bath-duration should reach 20 minutes at 30 C (86 F) with a carbon dioxide saturation of 40%.

- **Radon (Rn)**

It is known as the heaviest gas. It is colorless, odorless, and chemically inert. Radon was discovered in 1900 by Friedrich E. Dorn as a radioactive byproduct from the alpha decay of radium, thorium, and actinium.
It is considered highly carcinogenic and its therapeutic use is controversial.
Radon gas is easily absorbed through the respiratory system, the skin, and digestive tract.
Bathing in waters containing small amounts of radon gas is prescribed in Europe for a variety of problems like rheumatism, neuralgia up to diabetes.
Ingestion and inhalation is recommended as well. Twenty treatments are recommended as well during a 4-week program for 10 to 15 minutes at 35 to 38 C (95-100 F).

Other traces of minerals found in specific springs are:

Arsenic   (As)
Calcium   (Ca)
Iron   (Fe)
Lithium   (Li)
Magnesium   (Mg)
Potassium   (K)
Silica   (silicone dioxide) (SiO_2)

Arsenic containing spring waters are prescribed as foot or hand bath for athlete's foot and fungal infections.

Elemental arsenic was first described in the 13th century by Albertus Magnus.

Calcium was first isolated in 1808 by Sir Humphrey Davy, it is the fifth most abundant element in the Earth's curst.

Iron has been used since prehistoric times, it is the fourth most abundant element on earth. In nature, it is found in hematite, magnetite, limonite, siderite and taconite.

Lithium was discovered by Johann August Arfvedson in 1817 and is found in nearly all igneous rocks

Magnesium was discovered in 1808 by Sir Humphrey Davy and it is the eighth most abundant element on earth.

Potassium was also discovered by Sir Humphrey Davy in 1807.

For a more specific explanation, I recommend Nathaniel Altman's book *Healing Springs*. He did a tremendous job to categorize springs from around the world.

How, When, and Why to Use Plain Water Therapy

Disregarding the fact that there is never really plain water depending on its place of origin, I mainly want to explain the thermic reaction, the chemical reaction, and the autonomic nervous response triggered by a "plain" water application without mineral or herbal additives.

- *A thermic reaction* is accomplished by temperature variations where the water temperature determines the

- *Autonomic nervous response* through the stimulation of skin receptors. (vasoconstriction or vasodilatation)

- *A chemical reaction* occurs due to metabolic action triggered by a thermic reaction as response to hydrotherapy.

A cold-water application briefly increases the elimination of carbon dioxide (CO_2) and will then shift to a reduction of CO_2 elimination. Carbonic acid occurs by transferring CO_2 from the tissue to the lungs. By inducing hyperventilation carbonic acid is reduced which alkalizes the blood and consequently favors phagocytosis.

Alkalinity of the blood increases the action of leukocytes whereas acidosis inhibits those.

Heat applications lower blood alkalinity as well within the region of application. The increased respiration also causes the excretion of alkaline substances via the kidneys creating an elevation of urinary pH.

The impact of water can be further influenced by the amount of water (shower, gush, full bath, pool, ocean). A larger body of water determines proportionally the hydrostatic pressure and buoyancy effect. An additional mechanical trigger can be added by waves (ocean), jets (tub or pool), underwater pressure hoses or manually applied friction.

Galvanic electricity added to the water in form of a hydroelectric full bath or 4-cell bath has been a valuable form of therapy in Germany at hospitals and outpatient rehab facilities for a wide variety of neurological problems as well as post surgical therapy.

Whether the application of cold or hot is short and intense or long and moderate will determine if blood vessels contract or dilate. Partial moist heat applications like packs, wraps, and poultices create profuse sweating causing a loss of water, sodium, uric acid, creatinine, phosphate sulfates, and lactic acid.

Body temperature rises, blood pressure decreases (because blood is drawn to the extremities) and metabolism accelerates.

In a hot, full bath where the body is immersed in water, sweating is stopped; no fluid loss, or excretion of sodium or uric acid takes place during the bath. That explains why it is important to allow the patient to rest (wrapped in a blanket) for approximately 20 min. immediately after a therapeutic bath.

During this rest the patient may sweat so intensely that a brief shower might be indicated afterwards. So it is important to schedule sufficient time if additional massage therapy is indicated.

Since subcutaneous nerve receptors are extremely sensitive to temperature changes, alternating hot and cold foot- or arm-baths are the treatment of choice for neurological and circulatory problems.

Keep in mind that all hydrotherapeutic applications should be accompanied by 15 to 20 minutes rest, even the arm- and foot-baths.

The abundance of bath applications can become quite confusing because each form of bath has specific factors. The size of bath is determined by purpose and indication. (Partial bath, half bath, full bath.)

A partial bath is considered a hand-, arm bath, footbath, or sitzbath. For the hand, arm, or footbath there are several combinations possible because, generally, besides a local reaction there is also a reflectoric reaction calculated.
A partial arm-or footbath applied only to one side of the body creates a symmetric impact on the vasculatory system of the other extremity (arm or foot). This is referred to as consensual response where the opposite extremity reacts the same way as the treated extremity. For example, the temperature-increasing footbath creates a vasodilatation, which lets assume would be beneficial for the right leg, but the right leg has a cast around it and can not get wet. Applying the footbath now only to the left leg will create similar benefits to the right leg via proprioception.

If the patient has a general contraindication to a hot foot bath like a severe sclerosis of arteries throughout the lower part of the legs (feet up to the knee) a hot compress to the lower abdomen and upper thighs can be applied instead.

A half bath refers to a bath given in a small bathtub where the patient can sit upright, comfortably stretching the legs. The water level reaches the navel. Half baths are administered with or without extracts, hot, warm, cold, indifferent, increasing heat as well as brushing if additional circulation is recommended.

During a full bath the bather is generally totally immersed up to the head. The bathtub should be large enough to stretch comfortably. In cases where a person does not tolerate being immersed in water up to the neck, a three quarter bath with the water level up to the heart may be indicated. A cold compress placed above the heart region may also be helpful.
Full baths are also administered with or without extracts, hot, warm, cold, indifferent, increasing heat as fever inducing or fever reducing bath.

- Hot bath   38-45 C   100.4-118 F
- Warm bath   36-37 C   96.8-98.6 F
- Cold bath   13-30 C   55.0-86.0 F
- Indifferent bath 34.35 C   92.0-95.0 F

A constant temperature bath requires either a good insulated tub or the addition of warm water during the bath to maintain the desired temperature.

Another special form of bath is the quick hot or cold dip where the patient is only immersed in water for a few seconds.

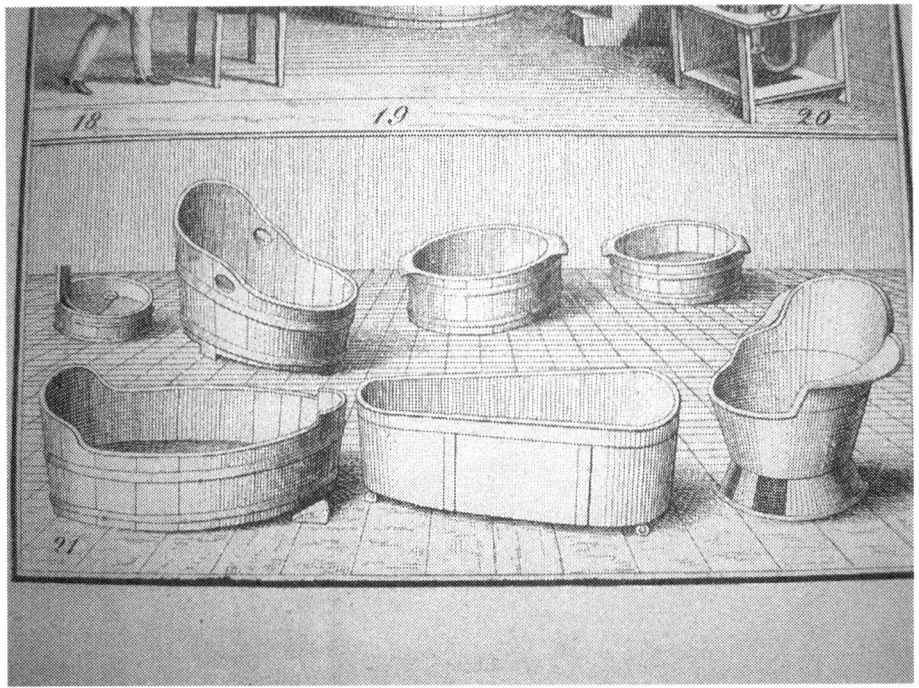

Teilbäder - *partial baths*

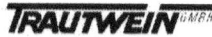

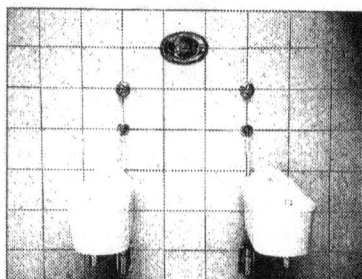

Wechselarmbad Modell Kneipp, Typ WA-WA-K
Contrast arm bath model Kneipp, type WA-WA-K.

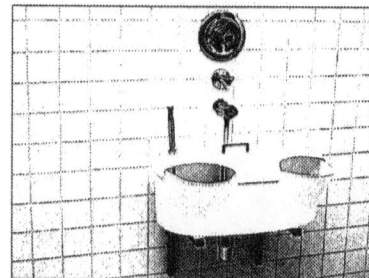

Hauff'sches Armbad Modell Hauff, Typ HA-WA-K für ansteigende Armbäder.
Arm bath model Hauff, type HA-WA-K for linear increase arm baths.

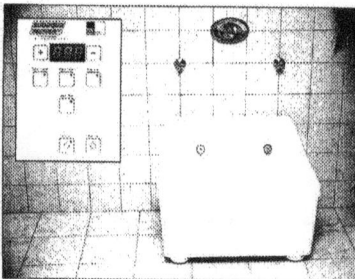

Wechselfußbad Modell Kneipp, Typ WF-WA-K
Auch mit Steuerung Typ WBS (siehe kleines Bild) Teile-Nr. ZT3019 für automatische Wechselbäder lieferbar.
Contrast foot bath model Kneipp, type WF-WA-K. Also available with control type WBS (see small photo) part-no. ZT3019 for automatic Kneipp contrast baths.

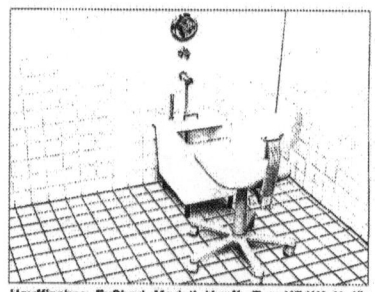

Hauff'sches Fußbad Modell Hauff, Typ HF-WA-K für ansteigende Fußbäder.
Foot bath model Hauff, type HF-WA-K for linear increase foot baths.

> **Farbauswahl nach Farbpalette ohne Mehrpreis**
> Choice of colour according to our colour chart without extra charge

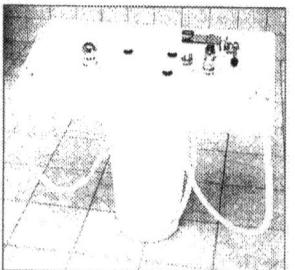

Dusche-Stand- und Wandkatheder sind in den verschiedensten Ausführungen, sowie mit und ohne Wechseldusch-Einrichtung und für unterschiedliche Wasserqualitäten lieferbar.
Auf dem Bild links sehen Sie einen Dusche-Standkatheder Typ DSK-WD mit Wechselduscheinrichtung.

Shower-desks and wall-mounted showers are available in different versions, as well as with or without change-over shower installation and for different water qualities.
At the picture on the left side you see a shower-desk type DSK-WD with change-over installation.

Vormontagezeichnungen und ausführliche technische Beschreibungen aller Modelle und Ausführungen stehen zur Verfügung
Pre-assembly drawings and detailed descriptions of all models and versions are available on request
Technische Änderungen vorbehalten   *Technical details subject to change without notice*

Trautwein GmbH, Denzlinger Str. 12, 79312 Emmendingen, Germany, ☎++49(0)7641/4677-0, ++49(0)7641/4677-70
e-mail: Verkauf@trautwein-subaqua.com   Internet: www.trautwein-subaqua.com

Partial Baths

- **The Cold Sitzbath**

Indication: create heat response in pelvic region, hemorrhoids, chronic consti-
pation, sleep disturbances
Prerequisite: body, especially the feet have to be warm
      Preheat bed for the rest immediately after the bath; heat pack on stom-
      ach is also appropriate.
Water temp: 15-20 C/59-68 F
Duration: 5-10 seconds

- **The Indifferent Sitzbath**

Indication: nervousness, sleeplessness, and hemorrhoids
Prerequisite: warm feet
Water temp: 34-35 C/92-95 F
Duration: up to 30 minutes
Patient's upper body is covered with a blanket. Bed rest immediately after the bath.

- **The Warm/Hot Sitzbath**

Indication: increase circulation in pelvic region, colon and kidney spasm, hem-
orrhoids, pressure headache
Prerequisite: warm feet
Water temp: Warm: 36-37 C/96.8-98.6 F
          Hot: 38-42 C/100.4-107.8 F
Duration: 10-20 minutes
Cover patient with a blanket during the bath except by spasm pains, a cold
quick rinse is possible if desired.
Bed rest

- **The Increasing Sitzbath**

Indication: increase circulation in pelvic region. prostatitis, cystitis, spasm pain
Prerequisite: warm feet
Water temp: start with 36 C/96.8 F and increase temperature every minute by 1
C/1.8 F up to 42 C/107.8 F if tolerable
Duration: 7-15 minutes
Bed rest

- **The Contrast Sitzbath**

Indication: creates equilibrium of circulation in pelvic region, menopause,
pressure headache
Prerequisite: warm feet

Water temp: two sitztubs required, Cold: 15-20 C/59-68 F
Hot: 40-42 C/104-107.8 F

Duration: Start 3-5 minutes hot and then dip for 20-30 seconds into cold, then go back to hot—Repeat 3x and end procedure with cold dip Bed rest

- **The Cold Footbath**

Indication: increase peripheral circulation, pressure headache, sleeplessness, nosebleed, increase vasoconstriction in legs
Prerequisite: warm feet (Do not administer any cold application if feet are cold) Preheat bed for the bed rest.
Water temp: 15 C/58.6 F
Duration: 15 seconds up to 2 minutes

Container needs to be large enough to place both feet comfortably immersed to "mid-calf".
Bed rest

Alternatives like "dew-walking", water treating, and snow-walking, which I will explain further under "Kneipp Cure", are also classified as cold footbath.

- **The Warm/Hot Footbath**

Indication: increase of blood circulation in feet and legs, post injury strain or sprain
Water temp: Warm: 36-37 C/96.8-98.6 F
Hot: 38-42 C/100.4-107.8 F

Duration: up to 15 minutes
Since the impact on the vasculatory system is similar to the reaction caused by the "cold footbath", it is left to the patient to choose the desired temperature according to individual preference.
Contraindication: severe hypertonus

- **The Increasing Footbath**

Indication: circulatory problem, chronic cold feet, rheumatoid problems, onset of a cold
Water temp: start with 34-35 C/92-95 F and increase 1 C/1.8 F every minute until 40 C, 42 C may be 45 C/104,107.8,118 F are reached
Duration: up to 30 minutes

Best use container or tub with overflow mechanism so warm water can be added continually or a tub with automatic electric temperature regulation. As soon as the patient starts sweating profusely, terminate bath immediately
Bed rest

- *The Contrast Footbath*
Indication: headaches, menopause, sleep disturbances, cold feet, circulatory problems
Water temp: 2 tubs required
        Hot: 38-42 C/100.4-107.8 F
        Cold: 15-20 C/59-68 F
Duration: 10-25 minutes
Place feet comfortably for 3-8 minutes in hot water then dip into cold water 10-30 seconds.
Repeat 3X start with warm and end cold.
Bed rest or exercise

- *The Cold Arm bath*
Indication: hypertonus, sleeplessness, increased circulation
Prerequisite: hands should be warm
Water temp: 10-15 C/46-59 F
Duration: 10-30 seconds
Container should be large enough to immerse both arms up to the middle of the upper arm.

- *The Warm/Hot Arm bath*
Indication: chronic cold hands, tingling in hands/rheumatic problems
Water temp: Warm: 36-37 C/96.8-98.6 F
        Hot: 38-42 C/100.4-107.8 F
Duration: up to 15 minutes

- *The Increasing Arm bath*
Indication: circulatory problems, frostbite
Water temp: start with 34 to 35 C/92 to 95 F and increase 1 C or 1.8 F every minute until 40,42 maybe 45 C/104,107.8, 118 F is reached
Duration: 10-15 minutes
Use container with overflow mechanism to allow continuous water flow to increase temperature or use automatic electric temperature regulated arm bathtub.

- *The Contrast Arm bath*

Indication: hypertonus, tension headache, cold hands
Water temp: two containers required

> Hot: 38-42 C/100.4-107.8 F
> Cold: 15-20 C/59-68 F

Half Baths

- *The Cold Half Bath* (half dip bath)

Indication: increase immune defense, due to sudden withdrawal of body heat strong stimulation of reactive heat production occurs
Prerequisite: Body must be warm/not immediately after a meal
Water temp: 15-20 C/59-68 F
Duration: 5-10 seconds!

- *The Increasing Half Bath*

Indication: bath to induce sweating at the onset of colds or flu-like symptoms/to reduce spasm caused by kidney stones.
Water temp: start with 36 C/96.8 F and increase 1 C/1.8 F every 5 minutes up to 42 C/107.8 F.
If profuse sweating occurs stop bath immediately
Duration: 30-40 minutes
-Bed rest-
While patient is sitting upright the hands have to be submerged above the wrist. Cold head compress might be indicated. Wash sweat from face occasionally
If patient sweats profusely during the rest period a quick shower afterwards is indicated (indifferent/warm-not cold)

- *The Hot Half Bath*

Indication: revitalizing
Water temp: 40-45 C/104.9-118 F
Duration: 4-6 minutes
Unlike the increasing half bath during the hot half bath hands are not immersed in the water

Full Baths

- *The Cold Dip Bath*

Indication: sudden withdrawal of heat, triggers reflectoric heat production
Prerequisite: body must be warm
Water temp: 15-20 C/59-68 F

Step carefully into the tub, not too quick, immerse down to the neck and remain 5-20 seconds.
Dry well, towel friction, get dressed and if possible perform light exercises to increase circulation

- **The Decreasing Full Bath**

Indication: fever lowering
Water temp: Start with individual body temperature to avoid sudden shock. Decrease water temperature down to 28–24 C/84.2–75.2 F within 10 to 15 minutes
Duration: max. 15 minutes
-Bed rest in preheated bed-

- **The Warm Full Bath**

Indication: generally relaxing, most suitable to combine with herbal or mineral extracts
Water temp: 36-37 C/96.8-98.6 F
Duration: 15-20 minutes

- **The Hot Full Bath**

Indication: stimulating, refreshing, has similar effects like the cold dip bath just without withdrawal of heat from the body.
Water temp: 40-43 C/104-110 F
Duration: 1-4 minutes
Immerse slowly, brief cold rinse after the bath possible if desired
- The Hyperthermic bath will be explained later under "Baths for Specific Medicinal Purposes"

Showers/Gushes

- **The Kneipp-Gush**

Long before Father Sebastian Kneipp, people had used cold and warm water to treat specific ailments locally. Water was poured onto to the body out of watering cans or hoses.
Father Kneipp refined those applications and developed a specific system which up to today is known as the Kneipp Gush (Kneippschen Gusse)
From an unnozzled hose, an almost pressure-less jet of water is applied to cascade onto the treated region. The hose is held 3 to 4 inches away from the body in a 45-degree angle. If a watering can is used, an uninterrupted gush needs to be assured. Keep in mind that for a knee gush 2-4 canisters of water need to be lined up. For a calf gush 6-8 canisters are needed.

The gush always starts peripheral (as far as possible away from the heart) on the right slowly moving towards the center.

Never apply cold water on a cold body!

- **The Knee Gush**

Begin on the back of the right leg, from the little toe of the right foot move lateral up to the back of the knee/remain a few seconds and move downward on the medial side of the right leg/leave the leg at the bottom of the achilles tendon and move over to the left little toe/there move up lateral to the knee/remain a few seconds and move down medial to the foot and begin the front of the right leg. Enter at the right little toe and move lateral just above the patella. Surround the patella with the water jet a couple of times and move down medial. Leave the right leg at the medial malleolus and move over to the left little toe to repeat procedure on the left leg.

The knee gush stimulates blood circulation and is known to prevent varicose veins.

- **The Leg Gush**

The Leg Gush is more intense than the knee gush particularly in its effects on the bladder, liver, and abdominal region. Begin on the back of the right leg just like the knee gush. From the little toe of the right foot move lateral up to the hip and remain there for 6-8 seconds to let the water cascade down the leg then move slowly down medial towards the achilles tendon and exit to move over to the little toe of the left foot/repeat same procedure on the left leg.

Now repeat similar procedure on the front of the legs, start again on the little toe of the right leg and move lateral up to the hip (approx. head of femur/slightly above inguinal lymph nodes). Remain again for a moment to let the water cascade down the leg and move down medial towards the medial malleolus to exit right leg and move over to the little toe of the left foot to repeat procedure.

- **The Arm Gush**

This is best applied on a seated patient. No cold gush if hands are colds or patient generally feels cold!

Start lateral on the little finger side of the right arm and move up to the shoulder, remain there for 5-10 seconds to let water cascade down the arm, then move down medial and exit above the thumb to move to the left arm and repeat procedure.

This gush can be repeated up to 3x.

- *The Eye Gush*

Patient leans over a tub or sink with eyes open. A hose is used to go around the right eye first 3x, then the left eye 3x with barely any pressure.
Indication: strain or tiredness of eyes, paralysis of eye muscle

- *The Facial Gush*

Gush starts below the right temple down to the chin and back up to left temple. Now the jet is moved across the forehead from left to right, back and forth 3x. From the right side start to slowly gush the face moving up and down from forehead to chin ending on the left side. Conclude by circling the face.
This can be self-applied by the patient.

- *The Ear Gush*

Plug the ear canal
Start with the right ear then the left. The hose is moved around the right ear to the right (clockwise) and around the left ear to the left (counterclockwise). Repeat 3x.

Gushes can be applied at warm, cold, or at contrast temperatures. Mostly chosen by preference of the patient.

Showers/Pressure Showers

In contrast to the nearly pressure-free Kneipp gush, the shower or pressure shower is pressurized. The water pressure is selected from 1.5 to 2 atm (atmospheres/= kg/cm^{2}). The pressure shower provides on top of the thermic trigger also an additional mechanic compound. It is almost impossible to create reliable pressures from a regular household faucet consequently these applications require professional equipment with thermometers, manometers, and warm/cold water lines. The motorized pressure system assures an accurate and uninterrupted application of the indicated water pressure.
The Kneipp versions of pressurized showers are known as "Blitz gush" (Kneippscher Blitzguss) where the water pressure inside the hose becomes slightly elevated through finger manipulation at the end of the hose. It is imaginable how many fluctuations are interfering with this form of application.

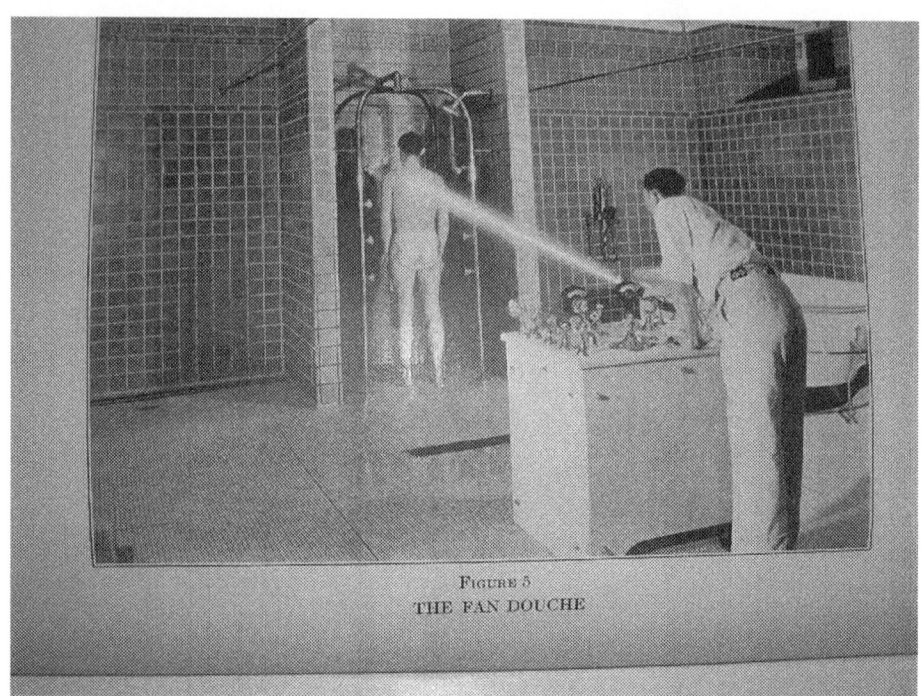

FIGURE 5
THE FAN DOUCHE

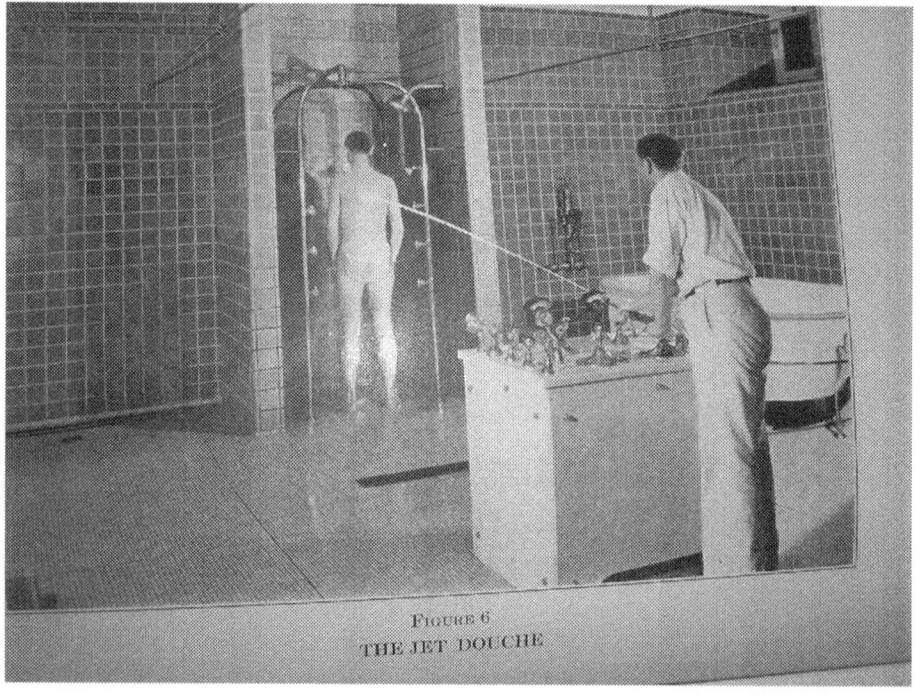

FIGURE 6
THE JET DOUCHE

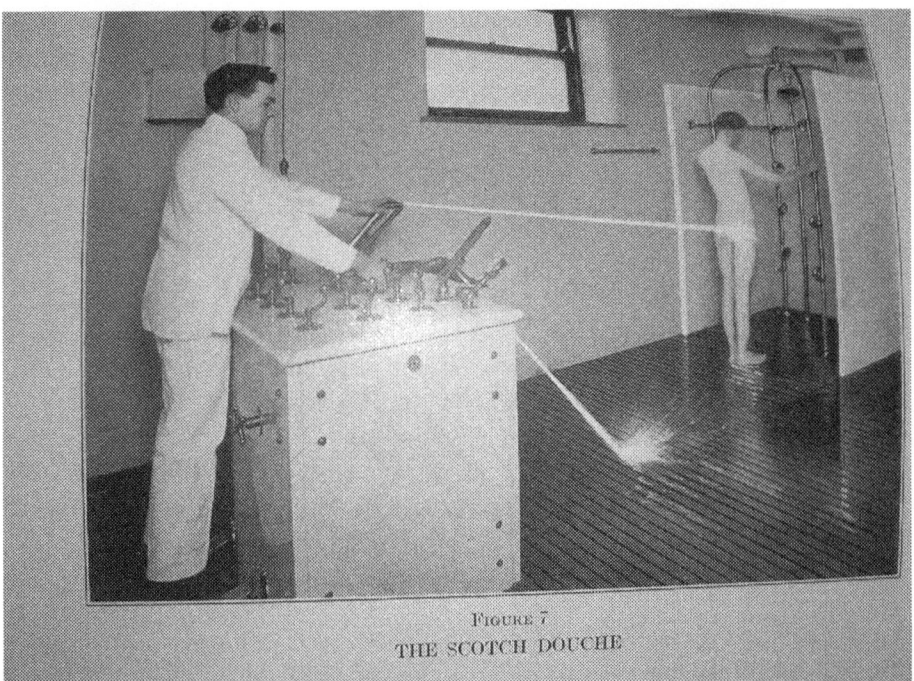

FIGURE 7
THE SCOTCH DOUCHE

- *The Jet Shower*

Water is applied out of a short hose or pipe of 0.5 to 1 cm in diameter. The water pressure hits the body straight on. The created mechanic response is much higher than in a regular gush therefore cold water appears to be less cold.

- *The Fan Shower*

If a split nozzle is not available, the index finger can be used to fan the water jet, but preference should be given to the nozzle to maintain a constant flow.

- *The Rain Shower*

is created by a showerhead, almost like a regular household showerhead except it is applied from about 1 to 2 meters distance in a 45-degree angle.

- *The Mist Shower*

Water is forced with high pressure through a very fine jet creating a fine mist.

- *The Scotch Shower*

is a form of a contrast shower using a fan or pressure jet. Starting with 40 C/104 F for 1 to 2 minutes followed by a cold jet for 20 to 30 seconds. Change 3x (warm/cold, warm/cold, warm/cold).

- *Underwater Pressure Massage*

Requires a specialized bathtub usually combined with galvanic and Faraday currents for hydroelectric therapy, which will be explained in detail later on.

The pressure applied through a hose is calculated in atmospheres (atm) normal range is between 1 and 3 atm but maximum of 7 is possible (atm=kg/cm^2). The patient is comfortably positioned in the bathtub with lukewarm to indifferent water. The hose is used under water only. The massage effect is differentiated by the size of nozzle used at the end of the hose.

Water, Steam, Ice, Mud, and Clay

As most abundant substance water covers more than 70% of the earth's surface and also exists as vapor in the earth's atmosphere. For therapeutic purposes water has been used for thousands of years in its natural occurrence as liquid, ice, and steam. However the icy stage of water should be used with caution.

If cold applications are indicated the best responses occur by using water or cold packs just a few degrees below the patients' body temperature. Historically the "coldest" natural applications documented, go back to Father Kneipp's "snow-walking" and his own winterly dips into the icy waters of the Danube River, which he did not recommend to his patients.

Waters in lakes, rivers, and wells always contain minerals dissolved from the earth, the same way like springs contain a variety of substances.

Different forms of soil contain specific enzymes, minerals, and acids determined by location and age.

There is a rapidly growing number of people becoming aware of the healing properties of certain foods, herbs, and waters, however very few are aware that the earth itself receiving its energy from the sun, air, and water is one of the most powerful healing agents.

In general mud consists of one-third soil and approximately two-thirds of water.

Soil is a complex mixture of inorganic and organic materials. Clay, silt, sand, gravel, and rocks are inorganic components. Detritus, organic wastes and a multitude of living organisms form the organic components. Soil is analyzed according to six general features:

- Texture
- Structure
- acidity
- Gas content
- Water content
- biotic composition

Depending on the "parent material", it may take 200 to 1200 years to form 1 inch of topsoil from hard rock. Softer substances like shale, volcanic ashes, sandstone, sand dunes, and gravel beds may be converted to soil in about 20 years.

Soils are classified according to the size of their individual particles ranging from clay (smaller than 0.002 mm in diameter) to sand (as large as 2 mm in diameter) and gravel even between 2 to 63 mm.

Soil is also influenced by its acidity level.

pH-
level
0 = Acid
3.5 = Sphagnum moss peat (Sphagnum moss is known to excrete antibiotics
and raise water acidity)
4.5 = Sandy soil
5.5 = Coarse loam soil and Sedge peat
6.5 = Heavy clay soil
7 = Neutral soil
8.5 = Fine loam

The therapeutic application of mud, peat moor, bog, or clay is commonly known as pelotherapy or fangotherapy mostly administered as partial packs or wraps. Moor or peat moor can also be applied as moor bath in a bathtub. For this purpose moorextract is commonly used which delivers the chemical components but not the specific weight of solid mud. A whole-body immersion in thermal mud requires constant supervision of the patient. Indications for mud and clay are rheumatic problems as well as dermatological complaints like psoriasis, eczema, dermatitis, and acne. A definite contraindication is pregnancy, severe hypertension, malignant tumors, kidney insufficiency, heart problems, and acute inflammatory processes.

All mud or clay applications require a quick rinse or shower at the end to remove residue. The mud bath (Schlammbad) consists of a soft mass of inorganic soil rich in silica. The peat bath (Moorbad) contains both organic inorganic matter.

Sand baths without the addition of water are naturally not considered hydrotherapeutic measures but they are also offered in some resorts where other baths are given.

Clay, which sometimes can be found in garden subsoil, about a yard deep can be administered like some spring waters externally and orally distinguishing it from other soils like mud or peat. Clay has the power to attract, absorb, or stimulate the excretion of toxic substances, it even has the power as bacteria destroying agent to convert contaminated water innocuous.

Clay has been used to eliminate the chemical chlorine taste in city water pipes. Inside the body, clay acts symbiotically and its value is determined by its physical-chemical domination. In general clay is known to contain the following oxides and chemical elements:

Silica   Calcium   Iron
Titanium   traces of Magnesium
Aluminum   Sodium   Potassium

But how many minerals exactly are contained in a typical clay compound only an individual analysis can tell. The montmorillonite clay from Nevada contains:

Arsenic	Chlorine	Germanium	Lithium	Palladium	Scandium	Thallium
Barium	Chromium	Gold	Lutecium	Phosphorous	Selenium	Thorium
Beryllium	Cobalt	Hafnium	Magnesium	Platinum	Silicon	Thulium
Bismuth	Copper	Holmium	Manganese	Potassium	Silver	Tin
Boron	Dysprosium	Indium	Mercury	Praseodymium	Sodium	Titanium
Bromine	Erbium	Iodine	Molybdenum	Rhenium	Strontium	Tungsten
Cadmium	Europium	Iridium	Neodymium	Rhodium	Sulfur	Uranium
Calcium	Fluorine	Iron	Nickel	Rubidium	Tantalum	Ytterbium
Cerium	Gadolinium	Lanthanum	Niobium	Ruthenium	Tellurium	Yttrium
Cesium	Gallium	Lead	Osmium	Samarium	Terbium	Zinc
						Zirconium

One of the "newer" clay bath creations takes advantage of the benefits created by the waters steamy stage. The so-called "Rasulbad" combines the old Egyptian technique of manually applied clay paste (covering the entire body) with an herbal steam bath.

Cold clay or mud applications are indicated partially if heat is supposed to be drawn out of a locally inflamed region.

The use of frozen soil is not recommended since it is not just impractical but also useless if not contradictory.

The effectiveness of peloids is mostly based upon their minimal heat conduction. It takes much longer to heat up a bucket of mud than a bucket of water but on the contrary mud cools off slower than water. Peloids retain heat much longer because of their pulpy origin.

Peloids and their geographical differences

Swamps are dominated by trees, marshes, by grasses, and bogs by sphagnum mosses and heaths. Bogs are most common in northern latitudes where retreating glaciers left moist, depressed land with poor drainage. Precipitation is their only water source. Bogs with a spring fed water source are considered fens.

Waterlogging lowers oxygen levels and slows plant decay. Dead vegetation settles and becomes peat, a precursor of coal.
Swamps and some marshes can also produce peat.
In some parts of New England, glacier melt kettle holes may simply fill in with peat and vegetation.
Central Ireland is known for its raised bog. Blanket bogs spread across poorly drained land, commonly northern central region.

Fango is an Italian volcanic mud. (Fango di Battaglia). It is soft, grayish brown, and of about the consistency of soft butter even equally soft to the touch.
It has no odor and is quickly removed after application by a warm douche.
Fango consists of 11 % combustible and volatile matter with carbonates, sulfates, sulfites of iron and lime, sulfates of potassium and sodium.
The application temperature ranges between 110 F and 125 F for approximately 20 minutes.
Fango conveys heat and retains it. Usually it is applied like a large poultice.
The effects are: stimulation of cutaneous reflexes, with dilation of superficial capillaries; increased activity to absorb morbid deposits; tissue repair.
Perspiration is promoted with a slight elevation of body temperature (2 F), subsiding rapidly after the application. The increase of body temperature occurs due to direct conveyance of heat to the blood.
Indication: subacute rheumatism, lumbago, rheumatoid arthritis, neuritis, sciatica, sprains and old injuries.

Mud Baths are generally prepared with saline or carbonated waters.
Most famous are the mud baths of Carlsbad, Bad Kissingen, Baden Baden, Leipsic, Vienna, Wiesbaden, Salsomaggiore, Abano Terme Springs, and Battaglia, Italy.
Germany has well over a hundred known "Moor Baths" categorized by mineral contents and recommended indication. In general, mud is made up of two thirds of water and one third of earth.
The therapeutic properties of mud are determined by the approximate length of its maturation because the prolonged contact between the soil and mineral waters can create a variety of chemical reactions within the mud itself, looking at the variety of mineral waters one will understand the abundance of chemical compositions in therapeutic mud.
The mud from Piestany in Czechoslovakia is famous for its high sulfur contents, which is accomplished naturally through the waters from a sulfurous thermal spring (152 F/67 C).

Specific mud is often collected from areas close to a spa or rehabilitation facility like in Calistoga for example where therapeutic mud is mined within the city limits. The specific ingredients of *Calistoga mud* are about fifty percent local white volcanic ash and fifty percent peat moss, heated by geothermal waters.

The *German "Moor bad"* (Moor bath) is a mixture of soil and peat also referred to as "Peat Balneology". The procedure to mix soil, peat, and water to create the right mixture for a "moor bath" takes about two hours. During this stirring process, the mud is also slowly heated to 40 C/104 F.

To fill a tub for a "full bath" approximately 350 pounds of moor is needed.

There are a few extracts commercially available which can just be added to the bath water mostly containing salicylic acid and essential oils but they are not equal to natural moor, which provides unique mechanic and thermic factors. In comparison to water as a good conductor for heat moor or mud does not transfer heat well but it distributes the heat more evenly deep into internal organs elevating the core temperature by about 1 C. This creates a variety of metabolic processes.

Deep Sea-Schlick is mud from the bottom of the ocean, rich in minerals and organic substances from decaying marine life.

Rehabilitation Centers along the Atlantic Coast of Northern Germany are famous for their Schlick-cure.

Most of the therapeutic Schlick is dug up from about 100 feet depth between Foehr and Amrum, two northern Atlantic islands, and than distributed to therapy centers nearby.

Before it can be applied Schlick also needs preparation in a "Schlickmuehle" which is best explained as thermic grinder where it is heated and remnants of shells and crustaceans are ground up until it is just soft mud.

Schlick also posses the unique conduction of heat typical for all other mud bath.

Contraindications: myoma, endometriosis, or acute inflammatory processes, severe hypertension, as well as heart problems.

Lymphostasis or Lymphedema because the specific weight of mud and the penetrating heat will create an additional stagnation of lymph.

If mud, schlick, or fango is administered as a partial pack it is usually applied to arms, legs, hips, or back as a 3 inch (10 centimeters) thick layer wrapped tight with a sheet and covered with an additional blanket.

The parts of the body not treated with mud are also covered comfortably with a blanket to retain body heat.

Paraffin is often used as substitute for real mud or clay packs since it also conducts heat very poorly but it is not recognized officially as hydrotherapeutic measure. The specific benefits are strictly thermic because it transfers heat slowly into the area of application.

Paraffin can be applied layer by layer with a brush; it can be administered as half-inch thick pack or poultice. Hands, feet, and elbows can also be dipped into paraffin and than be covered to retain heat. Paraffin is relatively easy to apply and it removes clean without residue it can also be reused if heated to 100 degrees C for sterilization.

Historically mud & clay have been used for medicinal purposes since the ninth century. Mud from the bottom of the Nile River had been cherished by Egyptians for centuries.

Mud and clay had been recommended in China against poison and pestilence. Documentations reveal the cure of stomach acid, colon diseases, as well as ulcers.

The specific healing clay promoted by Adolf Just in Germany is still available today as Luvos Heilerde.

- *The Loam-Vicar—Emanuel Felke*

Deeply inspired by Adolf Just's success Pastor Emanuel Felke focused on loam—applications, which brought him the nickname the loam vicar.

The Felke Loam Bath was introduced in 1912 in Repelen, Germany at his treatment facility, which was designed to house up to 400 patients.

At Felke's times patients had to dig a low trench 120 cm (47 inches) long, 60 cm (23 inches) wide and 40 to 50 cm (16-20 inches deep, which would be filled with fresh loam stirred into a mash with water.

Nowadays, patients are assigned to their own bath for the duration of their stay. The bath is still given for 30 to 45 minutes once or twice a day, for approximately 3 weeks. After the bath the patient roughly wipes off the loam and the remaining mud on the skin and is than briefly rinsed off with water from a hose. The patient should air dry if possible. The loam temperature can be cold, warm, or indifferent.

Felke was also noticed for his topographical drawing of the iris introducing mathematical exactness into iris diagnosis.

The Felke "Jungborn" (Fountain of Youth) is still "alive" in two natural health retreats in Sobernheim and Diez in Germany visited by thousands of patients each year. 3 weeks of Felke-cure with deacidifying mud baths and mud packs, combined with a vegetarian raw food diet are known to have lowered uric acid levels by 0.8 mg/di an average high blood pressure is reduced quickly to normal levels.

The detoxifying effects of mud baths and mudpacks have also proven beneficial for liver function (elevated bilirubin and Gamma—GT—indicators.

Felke's Jungborn was created mainly according to Adolf Just's Jungborn in the Hartz Mountains of Germany. Even Benedict Lust recreated a Jungborn facility in the Ramapo Mountains of New Jersey after visiting Just twice in Germany in 1906 and 1926.

Adolf Just's as well as Benedict Lust's facilities are not in existence anymore whereas Emanuel Felke's therapies are still applied and appreciated in Germany.

Despite the fact that Adolf Just's Jungborn vanished many years ago his Luvos healing clay is still available in Germany and its use is well documented.

Luvos healing clay is considered a terrestrial peloid which natural components are constantly changing but yet effective as remedy internally and externally.

Healing clay or Loess has strong absorbent properties it is formed through mechanical destruction of rock and other decomposing factors going back to the Ice Age.

Reference & Contacts

Emanuel Felke: Museum Priorhof
PriorhofsArasse 18
55566 Bad Sobernheim, Germany
ph. 06751-5232

Felkekur: *www.maasberg-therme.de/efelkekur.html*

Luvos Heilerde: Bund fur Gesundheit e.v

Healing Clay: *www.brgev.de/nl/heilerde.html*
           www.luvos-heilerde.org
           www.luvos.sagenet.de/services/html

LEVEL II/CHAPTER II

Complex Applications according to Kneipp

More than a century after Sebastian Kneipp's death, his Kneipp water cure is still respected and appreciated by millions of people all over the world.

In Germany, where it al originated, Kneipp water cure has been an integrated part to complement conventional medical treatments to prevent disease and speed recovery.

Spa treatments are part of a medical system aimed at prevention and recuperation. The "Kur" is purely for medical reasons and the specific treatment protocols are individually prescribed by a doctor located at the spa. The terminology spa refers back to the Latin "Sana per Aqua" ("Health through Water"). However in the United States "Spa" has a different image with beauty treatments, facials, weight loss programs, massages, and even plastic surgery selling the ambience and pampering. Natural hot springs in America are accessible to everyone whereas a European hot spring or mineral spring is diverted into "cure houses" or "cure partes" with access only by the cure-doctors prescription. Inspired by Priessnitz' rather crude cold water applications, the Kneipp cure developed into the Kneipp System augmented with other natural remedies turning into a philosophy for a botanical holistic lifestyle.

- *The Three Basic Components of Kneipp Therapy*
1.) patient
2.) temperature
3.) time

Kneipp individualized each procedure by adapting temperature and duration. He refused any stereotyped generalized therapy and rather focused on the peculiarities of each separate case.

It is important to keep in mind that for Kneipp "gentler" application meant shorter and perhaps a smaller areal but certainly not warmer.

- *Kneipp-Cure: Original vs. modified*

During the thirty years of experimenting and experiencing every single application on himself, Kneipp drastically reduced the recommended duration, this way he was able to moderate the intensity of his water applications. For example, before Kneipp, compresses and packs were recommended to be applied daily for three to six hours, the Kneipp packs are given for one hour maximum and only two or three times per week.
A cold bath was given for fifteen to forty-five minutes up to an hour, even longer, which Kneipp reduced to maximum of three minutes but often only ten seconds.

- *Kneipp's Synergistic approach to therapy*

Hydrotherapy as the center of the Kneipp Healing System was augmented with exercise therapy in form of walking, running, and gymnastics supplemented with various massage techniques and complemented by a diet in form of a wide variety of wholesome natural foods without one-sidedness or fanatism.
Herbal extracts in form of tinctures, teas, and bath oils as well as "regulative therapy" teaching the proper organization of daily life with respect to the biological balance between work and leisure, stress and relaxation.

The hydrotherapeutic treatment program includes ablutions alternating between hot and cold water or washing the entire body with warm water every 20 to 30 minutes to induce perspiration. Arm, leg, footbaths, hot or cold packs, compresses, affusions from an unnozzled hose or watering can followed by 10 minutes of exercise are individually selected and each application again is adapted to the patients' needs which may change during the course of their stay.
Each affusion is applied according to the individually prescribed sequence but all begin at the most distant point of the heart.
The contrast affusion begins with a warm spray right then left followed immediately with a cold spray right then left and repeat warm right then left. Kneipp's contrast applications always start warm but they can end warm or cold, determined by the individual protocol. For instance: warm/cold, warm/cold, warm/<u>cold</u> or warm/cold, warm/cold, warm/cold/<u>warm</u>!

A day at a Kneipp Resort may begin with an ablution of the trunk or a dry brushing of the skin followed by a cool after-ablution at 6 am. This may be applied while the patient is still in bed.

At 7 am. dew walking (walking barefoot in the dewy grass) for one to five minutes During the winter months this is replaced by snow walking for one half to one minute (again barefoot)

Stronger applications continue in the later morning like contrast footbath, knee or cold affusions as well as herbal baths.

The diet is mostly plant oriented, rich in vitamins, low in fat, whole wheat bread and fresh raw vegetables.

Breakfast: whole wheat toast, no butter and malt coffee

Lunch: vegetable soup, meat substitute, and baked potato, (followed by a rest)

In the early afternoon, sun and air baths are recommended followed by douches or baths.

For mid-afternoon, social hour snack, zwieback and sour milk or malt coffee is served. A nature walk followed by a supper and is concluded with an evening concert. If weather prohibits outdoor activities; concerts are replaced by health education lectures.

Even though Kneipp advocated a simple nourishing diet, free from all spices, and as beverage preferable pure water, but he did not object to an occasional glass of wine or beer.

But Kneipp's therapy does not end when the patient goes back home. Each patient is taught easy remedies to continue back home from hydrotherapy to diet in order to create a lasting sense of well being.

To show the comprehensiveness of Kneipp's therapies, the following case history explained in My Water Cure (1896/277) represents Kneipp's approach to strengthen the patient's entire organism.

"William, a boy of 9 years of age, had diseased eyes.

He could no longer read and scarcely distinguish persons, the poor little one was more than half blind. His parents had spent a fortune for the cure of these eyes but without result. The whole body of the child was just as impaired as the eyes. His hands and feet were always cold, his stomach without appetite, his body emaciated, his stature drooping and depressed Wretched are not only the eyes, wretched is the whole little man.

In 4 months, William was restored to perfect health of body and eyes. The little one had to take 2 warm baths weekly. 4 times weekly, I had a shirt dipped in cold salt water and put on him. He remained in it for 1 to 1 1/2 hours.

Moreover, I let the boy walk barefoot in wet grass or when it was raining. After the first 4 weeks, William took 3 to 4 baths of 15 R (18 C) every week: the baths were of only 1 minute's duration and always followed by exercise. They were continued for several weeks. The boy also washed his eyes twice daily with alum-water (a salt spoonful of alum in 1/4 pint of water).

As the body revived and recovered his health, the eyes, too, became better. At last they shone in the blooming face of the boy as if they had never suffered from the least disease."

Kneipp also recommended herbs externally in baths and internally as teas and tinctures. He substituted totally with oral herbs if patients could not tolerate the water treatments.

Even though the herbal bath was no invention of Sebastian Kneipp, herbs and flowers have been used for many centuries in bath waters before his goal was simple, he wanted to give his patients lasting relief. Not just a band-aid.

Patients who stayed for the Kneipp Kur also became educated about a maintenance program at home and to simply try to utilize the things within their reach.

If there is no therapist to apply water make due with an herbal bath instead.

LEVEL II/CHAPTER III

Kneipp Hydrotherapy at Home

The knowledge to use simple water applications and natural remedies to influence the body's system.

- Turn your bathroom into a "Health Spa" if you have a bathtub, a sink, or a shower with hot and cold water, you are more than well equipped.

A bathtub is nice but if you don't have one there is no need to call the plumber—learn to make due with what you have available. Remember simple—no stress!

Well correction, one little thing you may have to get is a five-foot hose. Since most American showerheads are wall mounted, simply unscrew it and attach that five-foot hose which can be used with or without showerhead.

Take your shower as you like but allow yourself 3 extra minutes at the end. Now use the hose if possible with cold water and pull slowly up your right leg from the little toe along the outside over the hip with the water fanning down. Then move quickly down the inside of the leg and repeat the left leg. Try not to splash. Repeat 2 or 3 times.

If you have time wrap yourself in a towel and go back to bed for 15 minutes without drying off-, but if you have to go to work just continue your routine.

If your body gets acquainted with this procedure you may get braver after a week and move the cold water hose not just up to your hip jump from the hip to the little finger of the right hand up the shoulder pull down on the thumb side across back to the leg and continue down, repeat on the left side. Do this only once.

This can become a daily routine I promise it does not take more than 3 minutes. This procedure can also be turned into a contrast-application: the cold water rinse is followed by a warm or hot water rinse and ends with a cold rinse again. These temperature changes increase circulation and release pressure or congestion in the head region. Definitely allow some time to rest after a contrast application.

A medicinal bath at home is generally a full bath with added bath oils or salts. The use of medicinal plant extracts became popularized through Father Sebastian Kneipp. Since 1891, the Kneipp Company in Bad Woerishofen/Germany has been manufacturing bath extracts based on Sebastian Kneipp remedies.

Essential oils are able to penetrate directly through the skin and are also inhaled during the bath.

> In order to create your own herbal or flower remedy for a bath you will have to brew a decoction best accomplished by filling a small sachet with your choice of botanicals.
>
> Place this sachet into a kettle of boiling water for at least 30 minutes then pour the entire decoction into a prepared bath.

This procedure is a little complicated and can be tricky at times because such extracts are difficult to preserve and need to be prepared fresh before each bath. Natural remedies containing tannins and salicylic acids like oak bark, oat straw, or even clay can discolor the skin and baths tubs so it might be a safer choice to select from a variety of standardized and preserved bath extracts.

It may be a little unfair to mention personal preferences at this point but I have used Kneipp remedies professionally for the past 25 years with good results and even remember my childhood where Kneipp extracts had been in use around our houses. However my grandmother preferred to go out and pick chamomile or peppermint for her tea preparations fresh, which was perfectly safe back then.

Medicinal plants used in teas need to be clearly distinguished. Leaves, flowers, and seeds are infused in hot water whereas roots, bark, and woody materials require boiling for 10-15 minutes.

The three most common formulations are:
- *Infusions* = flowers, leaves, and seeds infused in hot water.
- *Decoction* = wood, bark, and root extraction through boiling
- *Maceration* = extracts made with cold water to soften material by soaking or steeping.

Level III

MEDICINAL USES OF HYDROTHERAPY—COMPLEX APPLICATIONS OF NATURAL THERAPIES

LEVEL III/CHAPTER I

Baths with Specific Medicinal Purposes

At the beginning of Level II, I explained the general response of the body to water applications (thermic reaction, autonomic nervous response, and chemical reaction)

Medicinal bath therapy includes the benefits of all 3 responses in an individually prescribed order suitable for specific ailments.

There are two possibilities to create a chemical reaction:

1. Local surface stimulation triggers reflectoric release and excretion of chemical substances from the skin into the bath water.

2. Minerals, trace elements, and a number of other substances are absorbed out of the water by the skin creating a chemical reaction as well.
   (sodium (brine or sea water), sulfur, carbonate (CO_3), Carbon dioxide (CO_2), oxygen)

Temperature related stimuli create important reactions by manipulating the core temperature of the body. Which is maintained through metabolic functions and is regulated by physical and chemical mechanisms.

If the body is in danger to overheat from the inside (elevation of core temperature) it will start to release heat and sweating will result. (auto regulatory reflex) is now the perspiration process blocked like in a hot full bath consequently all other heat regulatory measures are blocked as well and body temperature will rise = fever.

On the contrary is the body threatened by hypothermia, it will increase heat production by elevation of metabolic processes like shivering to maintain balance.

The body possesses numerous defense mechanisms to gain protection against viruses and bacteria. To fight a major infection the body will deliberately create a state of hyperthermia to destroy invasive organisms, detoxify, or simply utilize a natural healing process. A state of hyperthermia is considered when the body temperature rises above 98.6 degrees Fahrenheit. Hereby the immune system starts to increase the production of antibiotics and interferon (protein chain able to prevent viral reproduction).

Hyperthermia can be accomplished partially to treat infection internally such as upper respiratory or externally for infected wounds.

The upper respiratory tract can be reached by inhalation of steam as well as local application of compresses on sternum or back.

Wounds on extremities are treated by immersion in "hot water" (as warm as tolerated)

In a systemic infection when a whole body response is desired a full-immersion bath, steam bath (sauna), blanket pack or increasing temperature bath (fever-bath) can be administered.

Hyperthermic applications in all forms are recommended for respiratory problems like bronchitis, pneumonia, sinusitis, as well as bladder problems, urinary tract infections, and cystitis.

- *The Hyperthermic Bath*

The Hyperthermic Bath or bath with increasing temperature serves the purpose of creating a fever-like elevation of body temperature. Temperature regulation through perspiration is blocked because the body is fully immersed in water except the face.

The slow increase of water temperature makes the Hyperthermic bath more tolerable and less strenuous for the heart and circulatory system than a general hot full bath or hot immersion bath based on the fact that the difference between the body and water temperature is minimized.

Water temperature: start with 35-36 degree C/95.0-96.8 F and increase one degree C every five minutes up to 40 to 42 degrees C/104.0-107.8 F.

Duration: depends how well the patient tolerates the procedure. **Bath needs to be terminated immediately if tachycardia occurs.**

Constant monitoring of oral temperature and carotid pulse required!

Pulse rate should proportionally increase based on body temperature. (at 40 C/104 F) 120-140 pulse rate per minute.

Does the pulse frequency increase too quick and the pulse rate reached 140 at around 38 C body temperature, the water temperature needs to be lowered to 37-38 C/98.6-100.4 F and cold compresses in neck and heart region need to be applied. This should lower the pulse rate quickly without decreasing body temperature.

In case nervousness and pressure around the heart occurs remove hot water from bathtub and add some cold water before patient is taken out of the bath.

Patient should rest for twenty minutes covered with a blanket.
Contraindication: Arteriosclerosis and circulatory problems of the heart. Risk of Heart Attack!

Cells of various tumors have a different stage of sensitivity towards Hyperthermic applications.
For instance fibrosarcoma cells are more heat sensitive than carcinoma cells, it is assumed that heat perfusion or elevated interstitial temperature creates the selective effect on a tumor. Whereas the blood flow to a tumor is considered the main determinant of selectivity.
It has been noticed that hyperthermia elevates the sensitivity of tumor cells towards chemotherapy consequently increasing the chemotherapeutic efficiency.
Hyperthermia leads to cell hypoxia and metabolic tension in visceral tissue, it is assumed that the antitumoral effect of artificial hyperthermia is associated with hypoxemia and pH decrease in venous blood creating considerable hemodynamic changes.
In regards of patients with brain blood circulatory disorders, it has been noticed that the auto regulatory reflex is triggered by the change in arterial pressure thus affecting the brain blood velocity.
Other studies have proven the immune system stimulating effects. While blood cells appear to drop immediately after a whole body hyperthermic treatment but increase within a few hours to a higher level with increased ability to destroy target cells. The elevation of interleukin-1 production has also been documented.

Hyperthermia is known to be a dangerous stressor, however the effects of whole body hyperthermic applications have been intensively studied since the 60's providing a collection of peculiar findings. (*www.43info.com/English/ Eng Articles/Whole body.htm*)

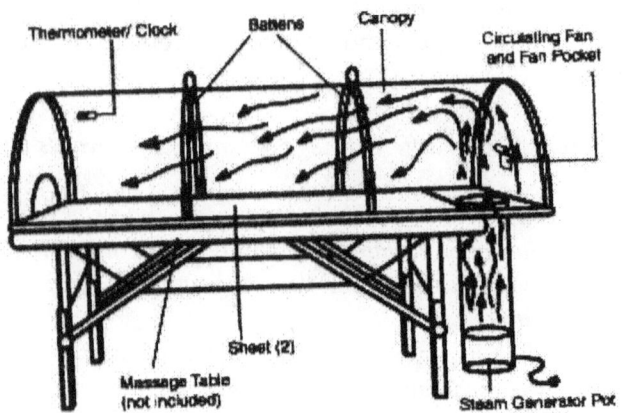

- *Steambath*
- **Steambath** or Sauna would also qualify as hyperthermic therapy. Turkish baths as well as Russian—Romanbaths have been popular in Europe for centuries. Steam therapy increases body temperature and consequently creates artificial fever (hyperthermia), which stimulates the hypothalamus, a gland that maintains and stabilizes normal body temperatures. Steam baths also stimulate the immune system through increased white blood count accompanied by antibody and interferon production.

Increased capillary blood flow to the skin removes impurities and stimulates cellular activity.

The cutaneous blood flow can increase between 50 and 70 percent.

The cardiovascular system is stimulated without elevation of blood pressure.

Pores open up and sweat glands start perspiration. Generally perspiration prevents hyperthermia by cooling the body through evaporation however due to the lack of evaporation in steam bath the body perspires without loosing valuable body heat = hyperthermia.

Duration: 10 to 20 minutes followed by a cool shower.

Steam inhalation has been recognized as effective treatment for sinusitis and other common cold symptoms.

Bronchitis, allergies, and asthma can be eased by relieving inflammation and congestion of the mucous membranes.

Steam inhalation also relaxes chest muscles and thus relieves coughing.

The sauna provides the same benefits as the steam bath but due to the additional dip into cold water or snow it offers also all benefits of a contrast treatment. Heart disease, severe arteriosclerosis, and diabetes are contraindications for sauna treatment.

- *Fever Lowering Baths*
- *The Decreasing Footbath*

Indication: withdraw heat, reduce body temperature in case of high fever
Water temperature starts for fever patients two degrees below body temperature to avoid shock.
Within 10-15 minutes water temperature should be slowly reduced to 28-24 C/84.2-75.2 F
Duration: 15 minutes maximum
Patients bed should be preheated, if patient begins shivering during bed rest, give hot tea to drink. Same procedure applies for decreasing half-or footbath.
Contraindication: coronary or circulatory problems

Notice the cold dip bath (15-20 C/59-62 F) is not recommended as fever lowering application because the sudden heat withdrawal triggers a reactive heat production.

- *Mineral Baths & Gas Baths*

Widely applied with synthetic extracts with good results if done right.

- *The Artificial Saltbath*

One 250-liter full bath requires 2.5 to 10 kg salt that equals an estimated contraction of 1 to 4 percent higher concentrations can create skin irritations.
Indication: improve cutaneous blood circulation, increase metabolism, strengthen immune system, rheumatism.
Water temperature: 35-37 C/95-98.6 F
Duration: 10-20minutes.

Salt baths are generally administered in therapeutic intervals with 10 to 18 baths per sequence. Baths can be recommended from daily applications to 3 x per week.

Patient should not shower or rinse off after the bath since the salt coating is supposed to remain on the skin. After the bath, the patient is required to rest for one hour (Blanket pack) and may shower than if desired.
Contraindication: heart problems

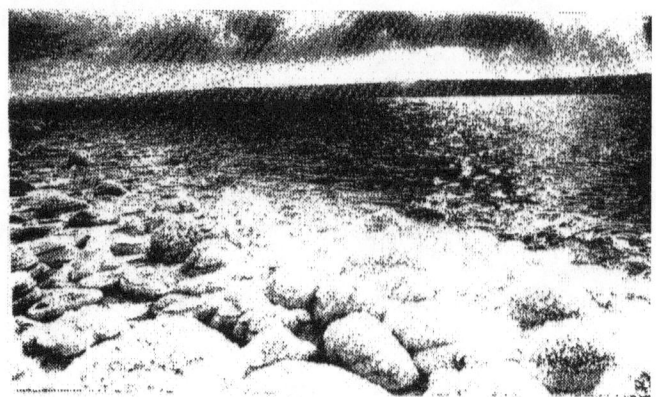

Dead Sea

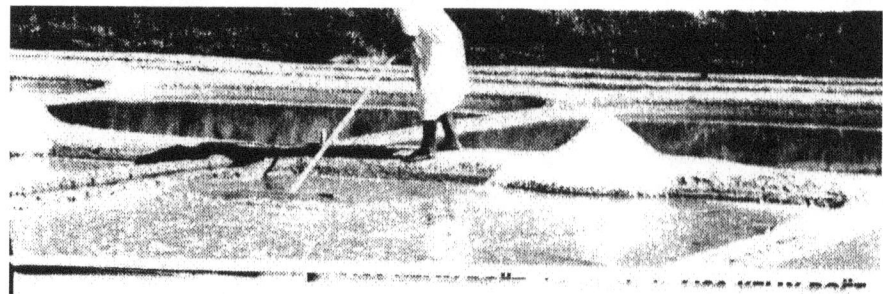

Sea Salt Harvest

- *The Artificial Sulfur-Bath*

    a) ready to use preparation (use as directed)

    b) for individual preparation (Hepar Sulfuris/Kalium sulfuratum is used) which has an extremely foul order and patients often object to that.
    In addition, the natural components of sulfur can leave black stains on skin and tub, the fumes as well corrode metal faucets.

Personally I recommend ready to use preparations, they are much safer to apply and bring good results.

Indication: improve peripheral circulation, increase metabolism and immune function. Rheumatism, joint, muscle, and nerve pain. Skin problems, bad healing wounds and ulcers.

Remove all jewelry before entering the bath!

Water temperature: 35-38 C/95-100.4 F
Duration: 15-20 minutes
General recommendation: series of 12 to 18 baths.
Do not rinse off after the bath, immediate bed rest 1 hour, shower can be taken after bedrest.
Contraindication: Arteriosclerosis, circulatory problems, heart disease

Epsom Salt is a chemical mixture of sulfur and oxygen formed into crystals.

Research has proven the occurrence of an immunohistochemical reaction of the epidermal Langerhans cells after a sulfur bath with 40 mg sulfur. It is documented that the function of the Langerhans cells is inhibited by 50% immediately after the bath inhibiting the Langerhans cell function. Sulfur is believed to have a direct anti-inflammatory effect on skin and mucous membranes.

- *The Artificial Moor-or-Mud Bath*
In contrast to the natural moor or peloid therapy which is generally administered in form of packs because of weight and mineral contents. The artificial extracts contain most of the minerals and acids but are supposed to be diluted in bath water.
Some of these extracts are well suited for home use or administered as medicinal bath in a spa setting. But keep in mind that even if the specific weight of the mud is eliminated which often plays a big part of its therapeutic value the minerals and acids alone can be quite stressful. Moor is a special form of nutrient-rich peat formed by gradual decomposition of organic material permanently submerged under water or underground protected from the decaying effects of oxygen. Providing the right climate and biological conditions it takes several thousand years to create this black substance. Most of the organic particles in moor are highly bio-available even the inorganic substances like iron, manganese, copper, and zinc are in "bivalent form" and small enough to be easily absorbed.
Use only as indicated.

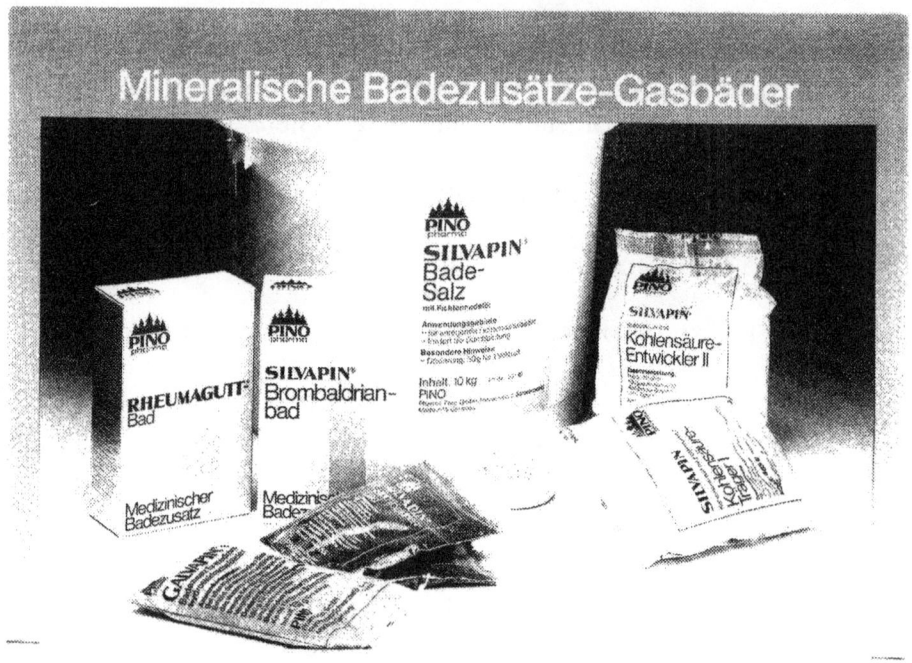

- *Gas Baths*
- *Natural and Artificial CO^2—Baths*

Indicated to expand blood vessel volume (vasodilator), improves skin circulation (peripheral blood vessels), cardiovascular disorders, and arthritis. Carbon Dioxide (CO^2) is a colorless, odorless incombustible gas formed by one carbon atom and two oxygen atoms.

It is naturally produced by combustion, decomposition or fermentation of carbon. Chlorophyll containing plants transform carbon dioxide into oxygen. As we inhale air we exhale carbon dioxide, but the human body is also able to absorb a certain amount of CO^2 out of the bath water via skin receptors, which then creates a cardio tonic effect on the circulatory system similar to digitalis, a blood pressure lowering component. These effects have been confirmed scientifically.

There are two forms of artificial CO^2 baths. One is considered chemical whereas the second is mechanic. The chemical product consists mainly out of Natrium-Hydrocarbon + a weak acid and is readily available.

Just use as directed.

The mechanical preparation requires special equipment mixing CO_2 gas (steel container) into the cold water with approximately 3 atmospheres (atm). The cold carbonated water is then mixed with the warm water in the bathtub.
This mechanical application creates almost identical effects like the natural CO_2 bath.

An easier system leads CO_2 through a hose directly into the bath tub from a CO_2 source, but it may create bigger gas bubbles and consequently poses the risk of inhaling too much released carbon dioxide for the patient.

Due to the large amounts of gas bubbles is the skin-water contact incomplete and the water temperature appears to be higher

- *Natural CO_2 Baths*
Carbon dioxide gas is rather expansive; the volume ratio to water is 1:2 (500 cm^3 Carbon dioxide gas = 1000 cm^3 water.) In compressed form (under high pressure) water is able to hold that amount multiple times. Those pressures can easily buildup under ground inside the earth and are often seen in thermal springs when hot water is propelled out of the ground.
There are also places where CO_2 gas is released solely. (Bad Pyrmont and Franzensbad/Germany) In the United States, Saratoga Springs in New York and Vichy Hot Springs in California are the most famous carbon dioxide springs.

- *The CO_2 Gas Bath*
Even though it does not require water, it still is considered part of medicinal bath therapy. These applications are well suitable in peripheral circulatory disorders, angiospastic, arteriosclerotic, and diabetic gangrene.
-Wet Skin reabsorbs more CO_2 than dry skin-
CO_2 gas can be applied as segment (partial) or full body treatment.
There is highly sophisticated and expensive equipment available but the old-fashioned electric light cabinet and a bottle with CO_2 gas can be absolutely sufficient.

The Oxygen Bath
In water, oxygen bubbles appear much smaller than CO_2 bubbles, which create a micromassage effect via the skin and consequently relax the autonomic nervous system.
Here also is a chemical product available which is safe and easy to use.

The air jet component, where air is supplied through jets directly into the bathtub via a pump is the more costly version of the O_2 bath.

- ### The Natural Radon Baths

Some hot springs naturally contain radioactive elements. We differentiate between radon springs with a minimum of 50 mache units of measured radioactivity and radium springs with a minimum amount of 10^{-7}mg/liter of radium. Radon is as radioactive inert gas with a very short life span, present in soil, rocks, and water.

In the United States, radon is considered a carcinogen and its use for medicinal purposes is highly controversial.

American homeowners are most familiar with radon tests inside their homes because radon gas can emanate from soil and rocks lying underneath a building or from building materials itself. Radon gas is easily absorbed by the body especially via the respiratory system, the skin, and the digestive tract.

Being banned in the United States as a health risk, European spas recommend bathing in water containing radon gas for multiple health problems like rheumatism, gout, neuralgia, even diabetes. Drinking water or inhaling air with traces of radon is known to have analgesic effects.

The most famous radon and radium springs still in use are in Germany (Heidelberg, Kreuznach), Austria (Badgastein) and Czechoslovakia (Joachimsthal, Teplitz).

The most unusual way of applying radon gas is offered in Badgastein, Austria where patients are transported over a two-mile stretch through a former gold mine.

With physicians on board, the train passes through four chambers containing radon gas with increasing temperatures.

Radon baths are recommended three to six times per week,

8 to 15 minutes at 35-38 C (95-100 F)

15 to 20 treatments are recommended

- ### The Artificial Radon Bath

In order to prepare artificial emanation baths, a concentrated radon solution is needed which is prepared in special laboratories for medicinal purpose.

Radon solution is only storable for 3 to 4 days; by day 4 the activity is already reduced to 50%.

Radon is soluble in water and oil, it is colorless, odorless, and chemical inert.

- *Detox Baths*

Substances are able to enter the circulatory system through the skin via diffusion into extra-cellular fluids, which then slowly penetrate inside capillaries and lymphatics.

Other parts of entry are inhalation and ingestion. Readily absorbable substances are oxygen, carbon dioxide, fat-soluble vitamins (A, D, E,K), steroids, plant resins such as poison oak and poison ivy, organic solvents like paint thinners and heavy metal salts (lead, mercury, nickel).

However the skin is not only the port of entry for many environmental toxins it is also an important organ of detoxification and elimination.

- Hot baths are relaxing, pain relieving, and assist to eliminate toxins.
- Moist heat applications cause profuse sweating, eliminating salt, urea, uric acid, creatinine, phosphates, sulfates, and lactic acid.
- Hyperthermic baths (fever baths) stimulate the immune system.

More specific are baths with baking soda and sea salt, epsom salt, hydrogen peroxide, and apple cider vinegar.

- *Baking Soda*

is strongly alkaline and can be used as full- or footbath to clear the body from low-level radioactive exposure emitted from tv-sets, computer monitors, x-rays, CAT scans, cancer treatments, or frequent air travel.

Two to six pounds of baking soda maybe used for this purpose.

- *Baking Soda and Sea Salt*

can be used one to two pounds of each per bath. This will help to detoxify from heavy metal exposure.

High saline concentrations make bath water denser than the body's interstitial fluids and toxic fluids are withdrawn from the body through osmotic pressure changes.

- *Epsom Salt*

is recommended as a general maintenance bath for hospital staff, computer operators, frequent "flyers", and people with exposure to toxic chemicals.

➢ Heavy metals: mercury, lead, aluminum, arsenic

➢ Toxic chemicals: automobile exhaust/carbon monoxide, solvents, formaldehyde, glues, Styrofoam, synthetic perfumes, printer and copier toners, art supplies, printing ink, household cleaners, residue from food and inoculations

> Low level radiation: TV, computer, medical diagnostic

There are different recommendations for the amount of epsom salt (magnesium sulfate) used per bath.

Profuse sweating is induced, the more salt the stronger the perspiration. One bath every three days is the maximum frequency unless otherwise prescribed by a physician.

Epsom salt baths should be applied as hot as tolerable for 12-15 minutes.

Recommendations vary from one to four pounds per full bath.

One to two pounds for general maintenance bath and to clear lymphatics.

Four pounds are recommended after exposure to radiation.

However documentations about much higher concentrations refer to baths administered in a clinical setting where 12 to 16 pounds can be used for the first detox bath and 8 to 12 pounds for the following sessions.

• *Hydrogen Peroxide*

The decomposition of hydrogen peroxide releases large volumes of oxygen (10 times the volume for a three percent solution), which in bathwater increases the oxygen availability to the body.

Concentrations of 3 %: can be used as topical antiseptic
                    6 %: for hair preparation products
                    30 %: industrial and laboratory use
                    90 %: rocket propulsion

Hydrogen peroxide baths are considered antiviral, antibacterial, and can also be used for chemical and radiation detox.

These baths are highly recommended as support during chemotherapy treatments. For this purpose six ounces of 30% food-grade hydrogen peroxide is recommended to be diluted in the bath water.

Caution: Do not have direct skin contact with this concentrated solution!

If standard 3% is used it will take three to four pints for a bath (1 quart to 1 gallon/4.3 to 8.6 liters).

Duration: 20 to 30 minutes

* Don't immerse face or hair! *

- *Apple Cider Vinegar*

baths restore the natural pH-level of the skin, which can be diminished by harsh soaps as well as frequent swimming.

By restoring the pH-level to a healthy acidity apple cider vinegar helps combat bacterial and fungal infections even vaginal.

The soothing effect on the skin alleviates itchiness.

These baths are recommended for general systemic detoxification as well as itchy skin conditions from poison ivy contact to sunburn.

Unprocessed apple cider vinegar is rich in potassium, phosphorus, sodium, magnesium, natural fluoride, iron, silicon, and sulfur. Other commercial vinegars make a weak electrolyte solution because of their low mineral content.

Two to four cups per bath are recommended.

As hot as tolerable for 15 to 20 minutes.

Level III/Chapter II

Specialized Water Applications

The world of protons and electrons is based on the fact that every atom houses two kinds of particles each being a minute charge of electricity, exactly equal in value but opposite in kind. (proton +/electron -)

All chemicals are equal in construction but vary in designation according to the number of protons inside their nucleus as well as the number of electrons circulating around it.

For example, an atom of hydrogen differs from an atom of gold only in number and arrangement of electrons and protons constituting each other.

The hydrogen atom houses one proton inside its nucleus and one rotating electron around it, whereas one gold atom houses 197 protons and 197 electrons of which 197 protons combined with 118 electrons form the nucleus, while 79 free electrons are rotating around the nucleus.

This comparison allows the conclusion that the entire universe consists of nothing but the two types of electrical energy (+ & -) in balancing proportions.

The human being as matter is built entirely by electrical charges in form of protons and electrons.

So we are really very delicately constituted electrical machines, built of and operated by electricity alone.

Free energy is required to pile up the individual atoms into a complete structure which is solely obtained from each atom's electron.

The varying current of electricity passing in one direction induces a current to move the opposite direction to create balance.

This game of proton and electron balancing is happening in every single cell exactly at the same time in each of the 38 trillion cells of the human body.

Blood capillaries are in close proximity to nerve fibers which carry off the negative current that is produced when oxygen gas gets dissolved in the blood while at the same time the positive current is accepted by the blood capillaries itself.

When the body is exposed to a current of electricity it will create a migration of ions inside the tissue and an resulting redistribution.

Pain represents the result of unequalized attraction and repulsion.

A) With electric impact

- *Stanger Bath*
    Hydroelectric Full bath

These baths take advantage of the high conductivity of water transporting galvanic electricity around and through the submerged body.

Galvanic electricity refers to a consistent direct current (DC) with constant intensity.

Many generators for instance as well as domestic or industrial power lines provide alternating currents (AC), a voltage that changes in direction many times a second. Charges move to and from instead of continuously in one direction while the intensity remains constant.

Electricity based on a constant direct current is known to increase reactivity and functionality of motoric nerves.

Peripheral circulation in skin and superficial muscle fibers is increased up to 600% and in deeper regions up to 300%.

The Stanger Bath is a combination between a 150-gallon bathtub plus galvanic electricity.

The bathtub has eight electrodes mounted into the inside walls, three on the left, three on the right, and one at the foot/bottom and one at the head/top. Each electrode can be charged minus or plus individually depending in which direction the electricity should follow.

Electricity always travels from plus to minus!

The original Stanger bathtub used to be made out of oak with portable hang-in electrodes, nowadays the bathtub is made of easy to maintain acrylic with built-in electrodes and absolutely safe control panel.

Indication: diseases of the central and peripheral nervous system, circulatory problems, ulcerations, rheumatism, paralysis

Treatment in general increases circulation and reduces pain.

Water temperature: 36-38 C/96.8-100.4 F

Duration: 15 minutes non specific setting flow from right to left (five minutes), left to right (five minutes), top to bottom (five minutes)

Exit slowly

15 minutes rest.
Intensity: on average 300 to 1200 mA up to maximum 3000mA.

It needs to be considered that approximately two thirds of the electricity is flowing around the body not directly through it, even though it is submerged in the water. However 100 to 400mA will travel directly through the body.
This may seem a lot but keep in mind that the direct amount of electricity is spread after the entire surface of the body in contrast to the two or four cell bath where the applied electricity full travels through the body as only conductor.

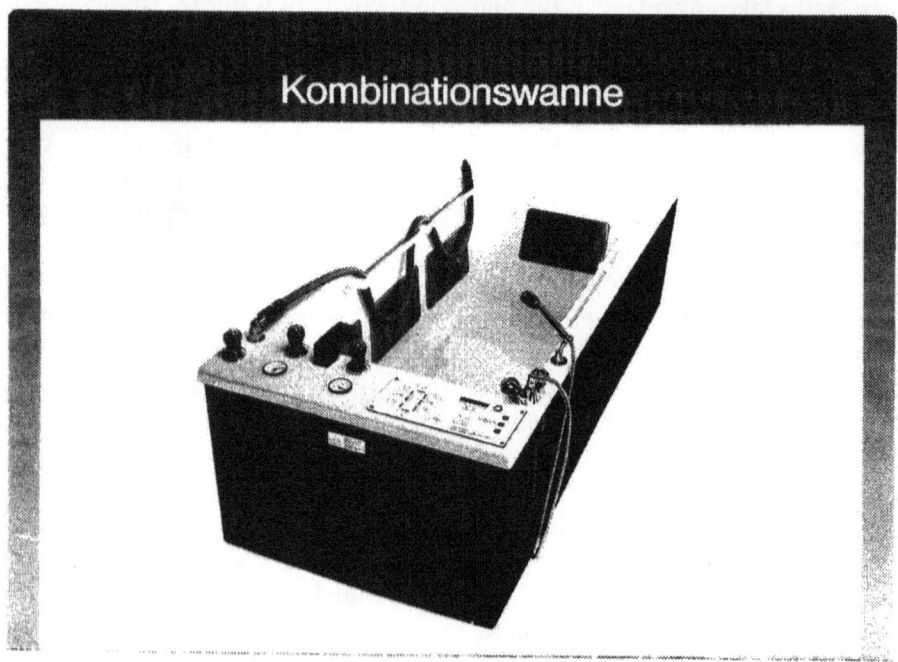

Stanger Bathtub

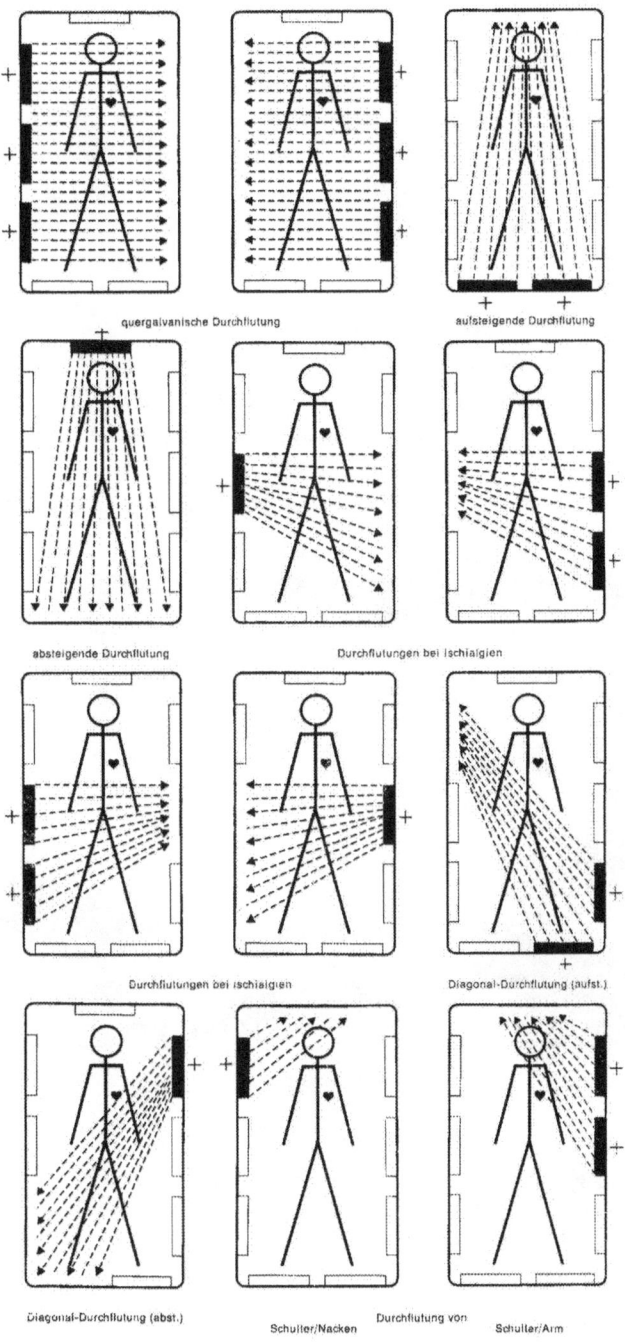

quergalvanische Durchflutung

aufsteigende Durchflutung

absteigende Durchflutung

Durchflutungen bei Ischialgien

Durchflutungen bei Ischialgien

Diagonal-Durchflutung (aufst.)

Diagonal-Durchflutung (abst.)

Durchflutung von
Schulter/Nacken   Schulter/Arm

- ■ *Stanger Bath*
- • *The 4 or 2 Cell Bath*

Refers to a hydroelectric partial bath consisting of two arm and two feet containers with separate electrodes.

Arm or foot containers can be used and connected independently. You may use all four or just two containers with the same principle that electricity travels from plus to minus but compared to the Stanger bath the connection or conductor between the containers is the body.

Water temperature: 36-38 C/96.8-100.4 F

Duration: 10 to 20 minutes

Intensity: maximum 80 mA

For the purpose of this bath, the patient only removes clothing from the extremities being submerged in water otherwise the patient remains dressed. A 10-minute rest after treatment should be allowed.

General Contraindication: metal implants, pacemaker, and inflammatory skin diseases

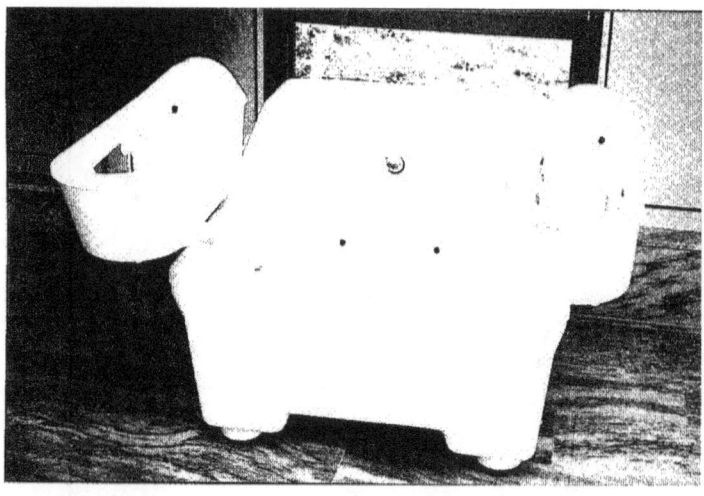

Four-Cell Bathtub-

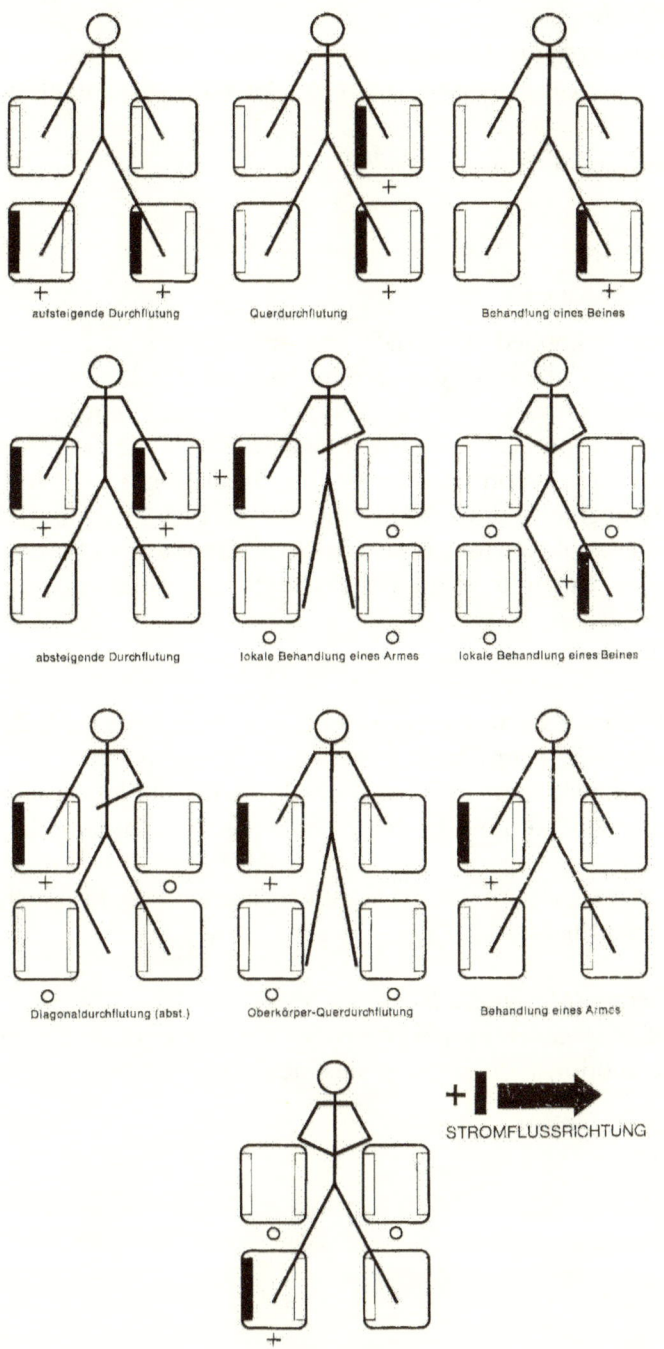

aufsteigende Durchflutung

Querdurchflutung

Behandlung eines Beines

absteigende Durchflutung

lokale Behandlung eines Armes

lokale Behandlung eines Beines

Diagonaldurchflutung (abst.)

Oberkörper-Querdurchflutung

Behandlung eines Armes

STROMFLUSSRICHTUNG

Unterkörper-Querdurchflutung

B) Mechanical Impact
- *Underwater Pressure Massage*

is a specialized form of massage therapy possessing physiological benefits of water therapy like:

> ➢ Hydrostatic pressure
>
> ➢ Buoyancy
>
> ➢ Temperature
>
> ➢ Force of Resistance

The treatment is applied in specially equipped 150-gallon bathtubs generally combination tubs which are also used for hydroelectric bath treatments.

Since underwater pressure massage is administered in warm water 36-38 C/96.8-100.4 F, it provides a systemic benefit. Beside the neuromuscular and central nervous relaxation a cardiovascular stimulation is triggered.

The warm temperature of the water starts to relax painful muscles and allows the jet of water applied with a hose to penetrate into deeper tissue.

Duration: allow patient to adapt to the water for five minutes before treatment of twenty minutes.

Rest for 15 minutes afterwards

For general treatment, start at the most distant part from the heart, the right foot while the patient comfortably positioned facing up.

From the foot slowly move up in partially clockwise rotation and pulling of jet, surround knee 3x and move lateral to the hip. Repeat same on left leg. Avoid varicose veins.

Move to right then left arm and have patient turn to the right side then left side in order to treat the back.

- *Water exercise/Motion Bath*

Water exercise is generally performed as group exercise in a pool setting whereas the motion bath is more specifically applied in a special butterfly shaped tub.

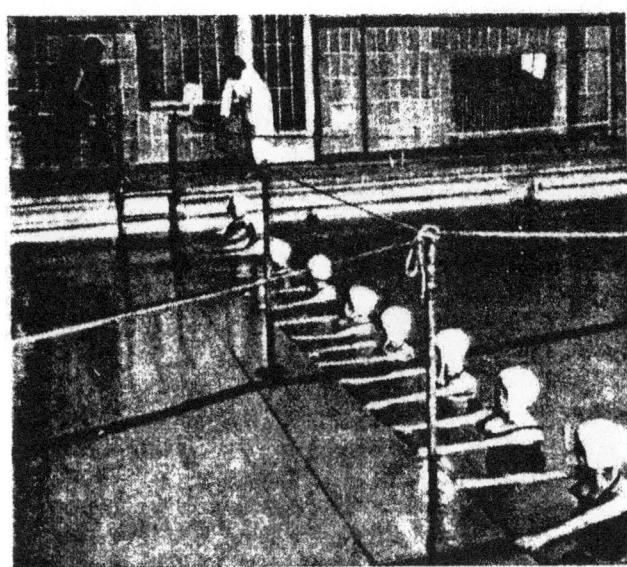

Abb. 63

Abb. 63/64. Übungsbecken aus Bad Oeynhausen (Frauenklinik, Prof. Siedentopf)

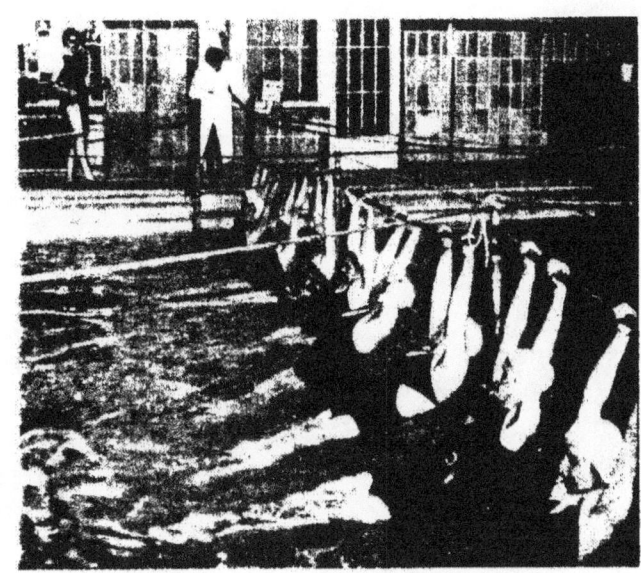

Abb. 64

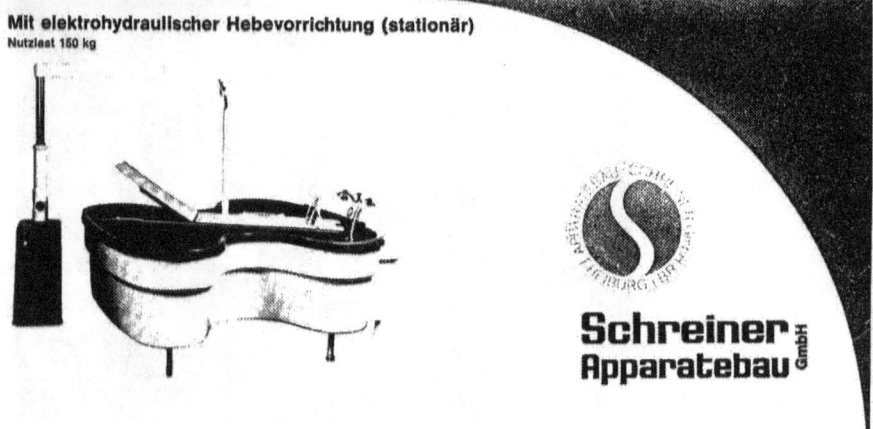

Schmetterlingswanne aus Kunststoff (GFK)

Bestell-Nr. 64212

Mit elektrohydraulischer Hebevorrichtung (stationär)
Nutzlast 150 kg

Schreiner Apparatebau GmbH

Butterfly tub?

With increased amounts of water the physical benefits of hydrostatic pressure and buoyancy are equally noticeable. Exercise, which might not be manageable for specific patients appear to be easy tasks under water. However only exercises performed slowly are easier, it becomes much harder if the same motion is executed quickly because of frictional resistance. The benefit of buoyancy is than replaced by resistance and harder muscle work is required to overcome this factor and the result can be muscle strain.

The buoyancy effect, which diminishes the impact of gravity, is mostly utilized while floating. The most therapeutic effects of water exercise is increase in muscle strength, mobilizing joints, reduction of spasticity, relaxation, improvement in balance and coordination because as soon as the body shape or posture changes, the water will fully balance it in its new position.
However, all factors of importance in general medicinal bath therapy do also apply for underwater exercise.
See Intro/Chapter I

Level III/Chapter III

Phytoextracts & Herbal Bath Preparation

Going back to Father Kneipp who did not exclusively recommend cold-water applications like Priessnitz, if indicated Kneipp ordered hot water treatments, which usually contained medicinal herbs for various problems.

The skin is not only permeable to drugs and toxins; plant extracts diluted in bath water can be absorbed as well.

It has been proven that herbal bath preparations enhance the skin stimulation. Pine baths for instance are known to increase white blood cells considerably.

Herbal bath preparations preferably bath oils have the advantage that they can be comfortably used at home. The classification of medicinal herb baths by indication appears to be somewhat difficult, as their actions tend to overlap.

Some times, simple preference is the indicator for selection. If you have three or four preparations equally effective for your purpose choose the most appealing, you may alternate, but don't mix.

- *Pine Baths*

Young shoots from 60 to 80 year old trees are preferably used since they contain the most active ingredients. An extract is produced in three stages:

> ➤ Distillation to obtain the volatile oils

> ➤ Extraction of water soluble constituents

> ➤ Inspissation (partial concentration) under vacuum to achieve a syrupy consistency

Three kinds of pine bath preparations are used:

> ➤ *Whole pine needle extract* from needles and young shoots, which contains volatile oils and 16 percent tannic acid or tannin ($C_{76}H_{52}O_{46}$), an

organic substance that is also commercially used to preserve animal hides and manufacture ink.

Medically tannic acid is used to treat burns because of its astringent properties.

➤ *Tannin bath extract* is produced from the bark and contains 28 percent tannin (tannic acid). This extract is mainly used to treat persistent rheumatic conditions. (Caution: strong skin irritant)

➤ *Pine wood extract* is obtained from the wood, it contains less volatile oils.

General Indications: skin stimulant, sleeplessness, rheumatism and arthritis as well as nervous and neuralgic problems.

- **Oak Bark Baths**

Oak bark does not contain volatile oils only tannic, which is measured up to 30 percent on average. Since it provokes a strictly localized reaction it is generally used as partial bath or compress.

- **Bran Baths**

Have a soothing (enveloping) effect on the skin and are generally used for acute skin irritations or sensitive skin intolerant to soap.

General Indications; calming, reduces itching, can be blended with lavender extract.

- **Lavender Baths**

Are considered beneficial for the entire nervous system, it is stimulating and toning.

Lavender reduces itching, swelling, relaxes and energizes as well established folk remedy, lavender is therapeutically one of the most versatile plants.

Some of the medicinal effectiveness is accomplished via the olfactory nerves influencing in particular the autonomic center in the midbrain.

- **Valerian Baths**

Has sedative and sleep-inducing properties; it can be combined with hops, which is also known for its calming qualities. It relieves nervous tension and headaches.

- **Melissa Baths**

Possesses sedative and relaxing properties which makes it suitable for nervous heart conditions and general restlessness.

It can be combined with orange and linden blossoms, which makes it more harmonizing, reduces stress tension, and anxiety.

- *Rosemary Baths*

Due to its camphor contents very stimulating, best taken in the morning. The transcutaneous absorption of camphor has been scientifically proven. One of the earliest plants used for food, medicine, and magic. Sprigs of rosemary were burned in shrines in ancient Greece to fight evil spirits.

- *Thyme Bath*

Mostly recommended as steam-bath for inhalation, the evaporating oils are beneficial for all spasmolytic and bronchiolytic problems, chronic coughs, emphysema, and whooping cough.

- *Camomile Baths*

Also known as German Chamomile is calming, soothing, and anti-inflammatory, it relieves the irritation of chronic eczema and promotes wound healing.

- *Juniper Baths*

The Romans used juniper for their "magic wreath" to ward off evil spirits. The bath detoxifies and sooths tired, aching muscles.

Glossary

1.) **Acetylcholine**—a major neurotransmitter found in the brain, where it has been implicated in regulating memory. It is also the transmitter, which activates the skeletal and smooth muscles in the body.

2.) **Allergy**—a hypersensitive state acquired through repeated exposure to a particular environmental substance. It is characterized by activation of the immune system and inflammation.

3.) **Ampere/milliampere (amp/A/mA)**-unit to measure the rate of flow of an electric current

4.) **Antibody**—the protein product of a plasma cell, which is capable of combining with the antigen that triggered its production. They can have multiple functions, but most often contribute to the elimination of antigen from the body.

5.) **Antigen**—a substance that is recognized as being non-self, and that is capable of eliciting an immune response. It is also capable of combining with antibodies and/or T-cells.

6.) **Anti-Serum**—serum containing a specific type of antibody.

7.) **Auto-antibody**—An antibody that attaches itself to self-antigens. Such antibodies can sometimes trigger tissue damage and specific forms of autoimmune disease.

8.) **Autoimmunity**—an immune response directed against a person's own healthy cells or their constituents.

9.) **Autonomic nervous system**—the components of the nervous system that regulates internal organs. It is comprised of the sympathetic and parasympathetic branches.

10.) **Basal Layer**—the deepest region of the epidermis

11.) **Cell-mediated immunity**—a form of defense characterized predominately by lymphocytes and phagocytic cells.

12.) **Collagen**—a protein substance in the skin and connective tissues (koila= glue, gen=producing)

13.) **Chemotaxis**—a process characterized by cells migrating to a particular site as a consequence of specific chemicals; eg., phagocytic cells migrating to the site of an invading pathogen as a consequence of specific chemicals

14.) **Cytotoxic**—substances that are capable of causing damage to cells.

15.) **Dermis (Corium)**—dense, fibrous connective tissue.

16.) **Detritus**—decomposed organic matter or biomass.

17.) **Endotoxins**—toxins produced by the cell wall of gram-negative bacteria (i.e., lipopolysaccharide). They have both toxic and pyrogenic effects.

18.) **Epidermis:** thin cellular outer layer of the skin without blood supply, but nerve receptors.

19.) **Epithelium**—cells covering external and internal surfaces of the body.

20.) **Epstein-Barr virus (EBV)**—a member of the herpes virus family, which is believed to be the causative agent of infectious mononucleosis.

21.) **Glucocorticoids**—Steroids that are capable of mobilizing glucose. Cortisol is the primary form produced in humans while corticosterone is the primary form produced in rodents.

22.) **Growth Hormone**—A protein produced by the anterior pituitary gland, which controls the rate of skeletal and visceral growth. It also directly influences the metabolism of proteins, carbohydrates, and lipids.

23.) **Homeostasis**—The events that enable the body to maintain a consistent internal environment.

24.) **Humoral immunity**—pertaining to soluble molecules such as antibodies.

25.) **Hypoxemia**—deficient amount of oxygen in the blood

26.) **Hypoxia**—deficient amount of oxygen

27.) **Keratin**-hard protein material found in the epidermis, hair, and nails.

28.) **Lymphadenopathy**—disease of the lymph nodes.

29.) **Lymphocyte**—a mononuclear cell that responds in a relatively specific manner in response to antigens.

30.) **Lympokines**—soluble products of lymphocytes that exert numerous biological functions during the course of an immune response.

31.) **Melanin**—dark brown pigment in melanocytes

32.) **Melanocytes**—found in the basal layer, responsible for skin color

33.) **Metabolite**—the altered product of a chemical reaction.

34.) **Mitogen**—a substance that is capable of inducing lymphocyte cell division.

35.) **Parasympathetic nervous system**—the component of the autonomic nervous system that functions to conserve energy and resources during relaxation.
Peptides—sequences of amino acids that can serve as hormones as well as neurotransmitters.

36.) **PH**—potential of hydrogen

37.) **Phagocytosis**—the internalization of pathogens into leukocytes. This process usually results in the destruction of microorganisms.

38.) **Pia Mater**—highly vascular membrane forming the innermost of the three coverings which envelope the brain and spinal cord.
Meninges are composed out of three layers: dura mata, arachnoid membrane, pia mater.

39.) **Pituitary gland**—the master endocrine gland located in close proximity to the hypothalamus. Its hormones regulate a large number of endocrine glands throughout the body.

40.) **Rheumatoid factor**—an antibody directed against IgG found in the serum of individuals who suffer from rheumatoid arthritis.

41.) **Sebaceous glands**—oil glands in the skin

42.) **Serotonin**—A vasoconstrictor found in many body tissues as well as the brain where it functions as a neurotransmitter. It had been implicated in a number of brain mediated activities including a form of depression.

43.) **Squama cell layer**—flat scale like epithelial cells

44.) **Stem cell**—a precursor cell that gives rise to the effector cells of the immune and other systems.

45.) **Subcutaneous layer**—(hypodermis/hypodermic needle) connective tissue and adipose tissue

46.) **Sudoriferous glands**—sweat glands (sudor=sweat, ferre=to bear)

47.) **Suppresser T-cell**—A type of lymphocyte that reduces antibody production by B-cells or the activity of T-cells.

48.) **Sympathectomy**—Destruction of the sympathetic nervous system, usually by means of pharmacological or surgical manipulation.

49.) **Sympathetic nervous system**—The division of the autonomic nervous system that is capable of mobilizing the body's energy resources. This usually occurs during periods of stress and arousal.

*Lewis, C.S.
Clive Staples Lewis 1898-1963
British author, literary scholar, defender of Christianity
Published ~ 40 books, major critical work medieval literature

*Because of the fact that the subject of hydrotherapy roots in German documentations, some words may have more than one correct way of spelling, f.i. holistic-wholistic

*Vasodilation refers to the relaxation or widening of blood vessels via nervous response. On the other hand, **vasodilatation**, maybe accomplished by induced medication. (Chemically)

Resources

- Curriculum for Specialized Hydro-, Balneo-, and Medicinal Bath Therapy. MCC 3508, MCC 3510, MCC 3509, MCC 3512, MCC 3513 by Carola Koenig, Provider No# MCE 468-05
- Library, College of Naturopathic Medicine Portland, Oregon

Special Collection

- Thilo vom Walde: <u>Vincent Priessnitz Zur Gedenkfeier seines hundertsten Geburbstags</u> (in memory of his one hundredth birthday) 1898
- Justus Verus: <u>Sebastian Kneipp Sein leben und sein wirken</u> (His life and his work)
- Dr. Friedrich Raimann: <u>Wasser-Heilkunde</u>, Ulm, Germany 1844
- Verlag Goebel & Scherer 1906: <u>Die Kneipp Kur</u> Harry B. Weiss & Howard R. Kemble: <u>The Great American Water Cure Craze</u>. Past Time Press, NJ 1967
- W. Teichman: <u>Wirkfaktoren Der Physiotherapie nach Kneipp</u>. (Special Edition Print)
- William J. Burroughs, Bob Crowder, Ted Robertson, Eleanor Valleir-Talbat, Richard Whitaker-Weather-Time Life Book
- Friedhelm Kirchfeld: <u>Nature Doctors, Medicina Biologica</u>, Portland, Oregon
- 1996. Castleman, Michael: <u>Nature's Cures</u> Rodale Books ISBN: 0-87596-301-3
- 1988. Gaia Original: <u>The New Age Herbalist</u> Mamillan Publishing ISBN: 0-02-063350-5 (pbk)
- 1988. Weiss: <u>Herbal Medicine</u> Hipppocrates Verlag   ISBN: 0-906584-19-1
- 2004. Medicines from the Earth: <u>Official Proceedings</u>
- 1941. Holder, W.E. (Fellow International Faculty of Sciences/London, England <u>"Electricity is Life"</u>

- 1976. Gillert, Otto: <u>Niederfrequente Reizstroeme</u> Richard Pflaum Verlag/Muenchen

- Gillert, Otto: Hydrotherapie und Balneotherapy in Theorie & Praxis Richard Pflaum Verlag/Muenchen

- 1996. Schimmel/Penzer. <u>Functional Medicine Volume I The Origin and treatment of chronic diseases.</u> HAUG. Germany.

- 2000. Altman, Nathaniel. <u>Healing Springs-The ultimate guide to taking the Waters</u>. Healing Arts Press. Vermont.

- 1997. Frohrlich, Horst, Hans. <u>The Nature Gardens of Sebastian Kneipp.</u> Sterling Publishing Co. Inc, New York

- 1976. Dr. Christopher, F, John. <u>School of Natural Healing.</u> BiWorld Publishers, Inc, Bravo, Utah.

- 1994. Feinstein, Alice. <u>Symptoms-their causes and cures-How to understand and treat 265 health concerns</u>. Rodde Press, Emmaus, Pennsylvania.

- 1991. Vries de Jan. <u>The Nature Doctor. A manual of traditional and complementary medicine. </u>Keats Publishing, Inc. New Conann, Connecticut.

- 1986. Huhn, Reiners, Knauth. <u>Physio-therapeutishes Rezeptierbuch.</u> Steinkopf Verlag Darmstadt. Germany.

- 2000. Dr. Peters, David & Woodham, Anne. <u>Natural Health Complete Guide to integrative medicine. </u>Dorling Kindersley Publishing Inc, New York

- 1977. Loffler, Helmut. <u>Naturheil Kunde Von A-Z.</u> Prisma Verlag, Germany.

978-0-595-36508-1
0-595-36508-6

www.ingramcontent.com/pod-product-compliance
Lightning Source LLC
Chambersburg PA
CBHW020433290526
45785CB00002B/832